D0820354

Key Concepts in Psychotherapy Integration

APPLIED CLINICAL PSYCHOLOGY

Series Editors:
Alan S. Bellack
University of Maryland at Baltimore, Baltimore, Maryland
Michel Hersen
Nova Southeastern University, Fort Lauderdale, Florida

Current volumes in this Series

A Continuation Order Plan is available for this series. A continuation order will bring delivery of each new volume immediately upon publication. Volumes are billed only upon actual shipment. For further information please contact the publisher.

Key Concepts in Psychotherapy Integration

Jerold R. Gold
Long Island University
Brooklyn, New York

Plenum Press • New York and London

Library of Congress Cataloging-in-Publication Data

On file

ISBN 0-306-45175-1

© 1996 Plenum Press, New York
A Division of Plenum Publishing Corporation
233 Spring Street, New York, N. Y. 10013

10 9 8 7 6 5 4 3 2 1

Printed in the United States of America

For Natan, Roseann, and Daniel

Preface

This book has been 20 years or more in the making. When I began my training as a psychologist and psychotherapist in 1975, the idea of integrating psychotherapies was barely alive, and far from well. My professors and supervisors seemed convinced of the certainty of their theories and methods. Clinicians and scholars who identified with any of the dominant therapeutic schools were intolerant of alternative points of view and were clearly unwilling and unable to converse cordially about any overlap in approach. Yet, my experiences with patients did not teach me the way to orthodoxy. If anything, I became, and remain today, puzzled by the ability of others to identify any psychological or behavioral event as proof of any particular conceptual system or therapeutic ideology.

A few years ago I had the good fortune to coedit, with George Stricker, the *Comprehensive Handbook of Psychotherapy Integration* (Stricker & Gold, 1993). This volume was one of the many indications that the field of psychotherapy integration had made it through rougher times and now had reached a point of "coming of age" (Arkowitz, 1991). However, the handbook raised many questions for me about the status and future of psychotherapy integration. The contributors all wrote worthwhile and valuable chapters, and I learned a great deal. But there was little cross-referencing in these contributions: It seemed that integrators of psychotherapy were not learning very much from each other. Instead, there appeared to be emerging a new set of sectarian psychotherapies that shared a common interest in synthesizing elements of preexisting treatments and theories.

Do we really need, and will we benefit from, a new group of therapies, be they sectarian or integrative? Or, I asked myself, have

I set out, with others, to add to the clinical Tower of Babel? Where was the larger view of integration in the field of psychotherapy integration? And in what language or metaphor can and should it be expressed?

This book is an attempt to answer these questions. By reviewing psychodynamic, cognitive-behavioral, and humanistic therapies with regard to certain key psychotherapeutic concepts, and then by looking at integrative contributions to the same variables, I hope to set the stage for a larger, more general level of integrative discourse and practice. In borrowing the theoretical framework of narrative from many disciplines, my goal is to offer one alternative for theory building that allows many models to be synthesized without preference or exclusion. The central point of this book is to redirect the path of integrative efforts in specific, and of the broader field of psychotherapy in general, toward the search for fewer and more powerful therapies. I leave it to the reader to judge the worth of this effort.

Acknowledgments

I would like to thank a number of people, without whose efforts this book would never have made it into print. Eliot Werner at Plenum, Alan S. Bellack, and Michel Hersen were involved in this project when it was just an idea. Their encouragement, interest, and editorial acumen helped to turn an unwieldy and cumbersome proposal into a more streamlined and reader-friendly volume. Mariclaire Cloutier and her staff at Plenum ushered the manuscript through the process of editing and production efficiently and painlessly. Many thanks are due to Margaret Ritchie for her superb copyediting.

To Gary Kose, Chairman of Psychology at Long Island University, I owe many thanks for good friendship, hours of good talk, and a great deal of professional support and freedom. Joseph Newirth, Director of the Postdoctoral Program in Psychotherapy and Psychoanalysis at the Derner Institute of Adelphi University, helped me to find the magic and joy associated with writing and being productive.

George Stricker, Distinguished Research Professor at the Derner Institute, was as always a source of collegial advice and encouragement. Able and invaluable research assistance was contributed by Annie Chanler, David Baldwin, Elizabeth Potter, and Isabel Sanchez of the Doctoral Program in Clinical Psychology at Long Island University.

Part of Chapter 1 appeared in an article in *Clinical Psychology: Science and Practice.* Parts of Chapter 9 appeared in earlier forms in articles in the *Journal of Psychotherapy Integration* and *Applied and Preventive Psychology.*

This book is dedicated to three people, who represent three critical elements in my narrative: the past, the present, and the future. Natan Sarotzkin, my grandfather, was my first storyteller and my most important caretaker. He taught me the value of the examined life and of caring for others and was a model of quiet courage and strength. Roseann Ungaro has shared and created a story with me for almost 20 years. She has been a better companion, lover, friend, and colleague than I could ever have imagined for myself. Daniel Gold is the future and the point of the story. Each day his tale unfolds a little more with great joy and energy, and with the promise of more magic to come.

Contents

I

Theoretical Foundations

1

The Status of Psychotherapy Integration

A BRIEF HISTORY OF PSYCHOTHERAPY INTEGRATION

The science and profession of psychotherapy has had a relatively brief but stormy history. The organized practice of individual psychotherapy, with all of its associated theories and controversies, is essentially only about 100 years old. During that time any number of psychotherapy systems, traditions, or sectarian schools have flourished. Like political or religious entities, these schools typically have scoffed at the ideas and methods of each other. Psychotherapists have always been interested in, and have attempted to utilize, new developments in the natural and social sciences, philosophy, theology, the arts, and literature. However, for the most part, they have refused to learn from each other if their ideologies and allegiances are different.

This trend of intellectual and clinical isolationism has been contradicted by an originally small, but ever-growing, group of scholars and clinicians who indeed have been able to cross sectarian lines. These integrationists have aimed at establishing a useful dialogue among members of the various sectarian schools of psychotherapy. Their ultimate goal has always been the development of the most efficacious forms of psychotherapy that are possible. The integration of therapies involves the synthesis of the "best and brightest" concepts and methods into new theories and practical systems of treatment. Psychotherapy integration is a subspecialty of the ongoing

3

clinical, theoretical, and empirical scholarship in the general areas of psychotherapeutic process, technique, and outcome. It is a specialization and a field of inquiry with a relatively short but highly controversial history. Psychotherapy integration is both a set of ideas and theories and a group of technical procedures and innovations that have arisen from such academic and scholastic pursuits. Since the mid-1980s, the investigation of such constructs and methods of practice has moved from the fringes of respectability and clinical awareness to a more legitimate and prominent place in the broader fields of psychotherapeutic research and practice. Signs of this new status are found in the existence of two professional journals devoted exclusively to research concerned with integration. Each journal is published by a professional society whose membership conducts integrated forms of psychotherapy and studies them clinically, theoretically, or empirically. Studies of psychotherapy integration have appeared in increasing frequency in other older and more mainstream journals as well, and the topic of integration has been either the exclusive focus of, or a major agenda item within, many professional meetings and conferences. The number of books concerned with psychotherapy integration has multiplied enormously as well. In total, it seems that, as Arkowitz (1991) announced, psychotherapy integration has come of age.

Such hard-earned and newly found maturity and legitimacy as a field of inquiry and practice do not mean that all questions have been solved and all problems resolved. As will be apparent in the chapters that follow, psychotherapy integration is an open-ended and ever evolving set of constructs and methods that cannot help but be influenced by new ideas and information.

The first studies of psychotherapy which today we may recognize as integrative in nature or intent were concerned with the translation of concepts and methods from some psychological or psychotherapeutic systems into the language and procedures of another. In the 1930s and 1940s, several papers appeared which took as their task the conversion of Freudian psychoanalytic concepts into the terms of learning theories. Originally, these writers were concerned with the relationship between psychoanalysis and Pavlovian classical conditioning. As noted by Arkowitz (1984), whose fine history of psychotherapy integration has extensively influenced this more concise attempt, perhaps the first paper of this type was written by Ischlondy (1930), whose work was expanded on by French (1933) and by Kubie (1934). French was concerned with the correspondences between the Pavlovian constructs of inhibition, differentiation, and conditioning and the analytic concepts of repression, object choice, and insight. Kubie's expansion of these ideas moved him to consider the possibility that such phenomena as conditioning and disinhibition play an important role in the relationship between the analyst and the analysand.

In certain subtle but important ways, these early pioneers in integration were following a trend introduced into psychoanalysis by Freud (1909). He had noted the importance of compelling the phobic patient to actively face the phobic object — a preview of *in vivo* desensitization — and also experimented with setting time limits on the treatment in order to promote conflict and to gain access to deeper unconscious material.

As learning theorists began to include operant conditioning principles and organismic and complex psychological variables in their systems, such ideas were applied to the dominant psychotherapeutic approaches of the era. In the 1940s and 1950s, such writers as Sears (1944), Shoben (1949), and Dollard and Miller (1950) recast psychodynamic and client-centered therapies in the language and concepts of reinforcement and of the complicated internally mediated forms of learning that had been studied by neobehaviorists such as Hull (1952). These studies emphasized the reinforcement value of the therapist in terms of shaping or inhibiting changes in inner states or in behavior and led, particularly in the case of Dollard and Miller (1950), to modifications in psychoanalytic technique that emphasized activity and instruction on the part of the therapist. Procedures that today are commonplace in cognitive-behavioral therapy and in many forms of integrative therapy were introduced by Dollard and Miller, including the use of homework, role playing, modeling, and active and graded confrontation of fearful situations and internal states. Wachtel (1977) and Arkowitz (1984) have noted that the work of Dollard and Miller was much more influential in general psychology and in learning theory than in psychotherapy studies, and that their direct impact on psychotherapy integration was not felt until much later.

Alexander (1963; Alexander & French, 1946) modified his psychoanalytically oriented approach to therapy by experimenting with active approaches to the induction of change that were informed by the then-contemporary learning theories. A point crucial to later developments in psychotherapy integration was his introduction of the idea that insight into unconscious processes often followed behavioral change, rather than exclusively being the antecedent to change. This move away from a unidirectional view of change was highly influential in the thinking of many later students of integration.

A highly important trend in the study of psychotherapy, that was occurring throughout the same period as the work just discussed, was the search for generic change factors that were common to all psychotherapies. Although not aimed at integration or theoretical translations in themselves, these studies were crucial in breaking down barriers between adherents of specific theories and methods. Among the more important works of this type were the comparative therapeutic studies carried out by Fiedler (1950), who demonstrated that observers were unable to differentiate between psychoanalytic, Adlerian, and client-centered therapies or to identify the therapeutic ideologies of different practitioners. Such research, as well as the investigations of Frank (1961) and London (1964), pointed to the commonalties between the variety of contemporary therapies and collectively became, with the works of other authors, a voice arguing for a nonsectarian and generalist approach to psychotherapy. These arguments proved to be extremely generative of the more specifically integrative work that followed.

The 1950s, 1960s, and 1970s were marked by the flowering of modern behavior therapy, with its base in learning theory and its powerful technology. The study of behavior theory and of behavioral techniques by the minority of humanistic and dynamic therapists who did not immediately repudiate behavior therapy led to important integrations at the theoretical and technical levels. In a parallel development, as behavior therapy became more sophisticated and more oriented toward complex clinical problems, certain of its theorists and practitioners came to look to psychoanalysis, humanistic therapies, and systems approaches for guidance, ideas, and methods. Some pertinent examples of these truly integrative studies include the works of Marks and Gelder (1966), Weitzman (1967), Bergin (1968), Sloane (1969), Marmor (1971), and Birk and Brinkley-Birk (1974), among many others. These students shared a concern with searching out the underlying theoretical links of and similarities between behavioral, humanistic, and dynamic methods. Workers such as Brady (1968), Birk (1970), and Feather and Rhoades (1972a, b) experimented with the technical integration of dynamic, systems, and behavioral methods within single cases. Increasing attention to the complex interpersonal transactions within the behavior therapy framework led certain behavioral workers toward the dynamic, humanistic, and interpersonal camps, as did the increasing emphasis within behavior therapy on covert cognitive and affective processes. An important measure of integration from a behavioral vantage point was announced by the publication of *Clinical Behavior Therapy* (1976) by Goldfried and Davison, who acknowledged the utility of, and the need for, concepts and methods drawn from other systems of therapy.

If the history of developments in psychotherapy integration has a single watershed moment, it may be the publication of Wachtel's *Psychoanalysis and Behavior Therapy* (1977), a volume that remains the most frequently cited work in psychotherapy integration and has served as a model of integration at both a theoretical and a technical level. Wachtel offered a theory of personality and psychopathology that fully integrated critical aspects of dynamic and behavioral theory into a unique and synergistic model. Just as important, this new and integrative theory also allowed interventions from a broad range of positions to be utilized clinically and in a way that was predictable and comprehensible.

The late 1970s, the 1980s, and the early 1990s have been marked by an explosion of integrative works, and by impassioned debate about the possibility and advisability of integrative efforts. Of particular note during this period was the collection of dialogues between supporters and opponents of psychotherapy integration that was compiled by Arkowitz and Messer (1984). Although this volume must clearly be taken as an argument for integration, in fairness it should be noted that among the critics and opponents of psychotherapy integration have been some leading authorities on psychotherapy, including Wolpe (1984), Franks (1984), Messer and Winokur (1984), and Lazarus (1989). A final sign of the evolving maturity of psychotherapy integration in the 1990s was the almost simultaneous publication of two handbooks that collected the work of the major contributors in single volume sources (Norcross & Goldfried, 1992; Stricker & Gold, 1993). Readers who desire a more extensive discussion of the history of psychotherapy integration are referred to the excellent works by Arkowitz (1984) and Goldfried and Newman (1992).

THE NEED FOR AN INTEGRATED PSYCHOTHERAPY

Psychotherapy integration came into its own in the 1980s, and entered the 1990s as a vital area of study and of clinical progress within the broader field of psychotherapy. The sustained flowering of interest in integration is the result of any number of clinical, scientific, professional, and socioeconomic factors that are having an impact, and will continue to do so, on psychotherapy and its practitioners. Norcross and Newman (1992) identified eight interacting variables that have encouraged this growth, including:

1. The enormous expansion in the number of separate psychotherapies.
2. The failure of any single therapy or group of therapies to demonstrate remarkably superior efficacy.
3. The correlated lack of success of any theory to adequately explain and predict pathology or personality and behavioral change.
4. The growth in the number and importance of shorter term, focused psychotherapies.
5. Greater communication between clinicians and scholars that has resulted in an increased willingness to, and opportunity for, therapeutic experimentation.
6. The intrusion into the consulting room of the realities of limited socioeconomic support by third parties for traditional, long-term psychotherapies. This has been accompanied by an increased demand for accountability and documentation of the effectiveness of all medical and psychological therapies.
7. The identification of certain common factors in all psychotherapies that are related to successful outcome.
8. The development of professional organizations, networks, conferences, and journals that are dedicated to the discussion and study of psychotherapy integration.

The broader discipline of academic psychology has undergone many theoretical and methodological changes in recent times as well, adding broadly to an environment in which integration is admired and encouraged. More narrowly, integration has been supported by the ascendance of cognitive and information-processing theories in general psychology, and by a movement toward a synthesis of process and outcome positions in psychology and in psychotherapy (Gold, 1995; Orlinsky, Grawe, & Parks, 1994). Additionally, several of the more influential schools of psychotherapy, including psychoanalysis, client, centered therapy, and behavior therapy, have aged and matured as each has produced many generations of students and practitioners. Each new cohort has had a greater opportunity to be influenced by, and to influence, its counterparts and is further removed from the dogmatism, zeal, and xenophobic avoidance of earlier generations.

Underlying all of the past and present interest in psychotherapy integration is one central concern: the construction of the most efficacious theory and method of psychotherapy possible. As it has proved impossible to point out the winner of the psychotherapy success sweepstakes, it also has become very clear that most established forms of therapy are helpful to some significant percentage of patients (Luborsky, 1995). The fact that no single form of psychotherapy can be demonstrated to be effective with all problems and for all persons has generated a number of directions of study in the psychotherapy literature. Those therapists who are committed to a single method have expanded those systems from within, preserving the unique strengths of their system while adding ideas and techniques that are expansions of the theory and method that are unique to that approach.

Students of integration hope to promote a synergy of the more potent components of the various sectarian psychotherapies by combining them technically and conceptually. This difference between expanded sectarian systems and integrative systems is very important. Expansion of existing models involves attention to nuance and detail, as well as the refinement of existing theories and techniques. However, these modifications are suggestive of what Kuhn (1962) called *paradigm expansion,* a process that he suggested has more to do with the preservation of a given theory than with the search for new knowledge. Proponents of integration suggest that each sectarian model of therapy is limited to some degree by its ideology and methodology. These limitations are most apparent in the fact that all single systems of therapy omit several important components of psychological change while over-emphasizing others (see Chapter 3). Integration allows the inclusion of the most potent change principles, techniques, and ideas, without concern for the violation of the ideological norms or group beliefs that have trapped most traditional therapies in their respective states of isolation. In Kuhn's (1962) terms, psychotherapy integration reflects the exhaustion of existing paradigms. An example of a scientific or clinical revolution, it has resulted in the possibility of truly new ways of understanding personality and psychopathology, and in original, creative, and more powerful clinical procedures.

Any number of cultural and historical factors have also contributed to the emergence of integrative psychotherapeutic approaches at times (Gold, 1993b). In the last 30 years, Western culture has assimilated new ideas that have challenged former paradigms at an extraordinary rate and degree. The physical and social sciences, philosophy, and theology have revised our understanding of the world and the place of humanity and have in many ways moved away from certainty to relativistic theories that are more Eastern in content and outlook. At the same time, a series of cultural upheavals — including the Vietnam war, the sexual revolution, the civil rights movement and its aftermath of chronic ethnic and racial tension, the rise of feminism and of the gay rights movement, ongoing economic and environmental crises, the fall of the Soviet Union, and the AIDS epidemic (to offer a very selective list) — have undermined the ability of many, whether in psychotherapy or not, and without to believe in a sectarian model of behavior and of treatment. As belief in authority and in absolute models of knowing is eroded, a certain sector of the populace turns to fundamentalist belief systems and practices. Others embrace the best of previously competitive theories and techniques in order to move ahead. It is perhaps to the latter group that integrative psychotherapists belong.

In the midst of this unprecedented development and progress, however, there does lurk a potentially serious problem. The movement toward the integration of psychotherapies may revitalize and elevate the field of psychotherapy, or it may add seriously to its bifurcation and disintegration. More specifically, the proliferation of dozens or scores of innovative, integrative treatments and theories may cause the number of idiosyncratic, personalized, and inadequately tested therapies to burgeon out of control. For example, consider two edited handbooks concerning psychotherapy integration (Norcross & Goldfried, 1992; Stricker & Gold, 1993). These volumes contain a generous representation of the important work in this field and, together, offer the reader over 30 new forms of integrative psychotherapy! While the reader of these contributions, and of others in the integration literature, will find considerable cross referencing between them, it is also apparent that each author thinks that his or her therapy is unusual and important.

Can psychotherapy integration survive an endless proliferation of systems and methods? Does such unchecked growth and the ongoing introduction of new models of therapy really serve any purpose other than enhancing the self-esteem of the creators of such systems? Probably not. It is not the intent of this book to designate one of these many integrative contributions the model or "best" one. Rather, this volume is an attempt to establish a backbone for further integrations by pulling together into one basic system some of the key findings and contributions made by integrative writers. This tentative synthesis or metaintegration, then, may organize and provide guiding parameters for further work by providing current and future students of integrative therapy a foundation of agreed-upon and accepted knowledge.

THE MODES OF PSYCHOTHERAPY INTEGRATION

There exist three generally accepted ways in which the methods and concepts of two or more schools of psychotherapy may be combined or synthesized. These modes differ from each other with regard to the hypothesized point at which the component therapies meet and meld with each other. They are also different in terms of the respective emphasis placed at each level on technique, change factors, or broader theory (Norcross & Newman, 1992).

The three most commonly discussed forms of integration are *technical eclecticism,* the *common-factors* approach, and *theoretical integration.* The discussion that follows defines and describes this trio of integrative modes.

Technical eclecticism is the most clinical and technically oriented form of psychotherapy integration. Techniques and interventions drawn from two or more psychotherapeutic systems are applied systematically and sequentially. The series of linked interventions usually follows a comprehensive assessment of the patient. This assessment allows target problems to be identified and identifies the relationships between the different problems, strengths, and cognitive, affective, and interpersonal characteristics of the patient. Techniques are chosen on the basis of the best clinical match to the needs of the patient, as guided by clinical knowledge and by research findings. Technical eclecticism need not be guided by an original or integrative theory of personality or of psychopathology. Instead, it usually is based on existing theories and goes beyond this conceptual foundation on a case-by-case clinical basis, by adding new techniques and clinical strategies as they are needed.

The common-factors approach to integration stems from the assumption that all effective methods of psychotherapy share to some degree certain critical, curative factors. Common-factors approaches start from the attempt to identify the specific effective ingredients of any group of therapies. This effort is followed by an exploration of how particular interventions and psychotherapeutic interactions promote and contain those ingredients. The integrative therapies that result from this process are structured around the goal of maximizing the patient's exposure to the unique combination of therapeutic factors that will best ameliorate his or her problems.

The search for common curative factors in cross-sectional studies of psychotherapy has a long and distinguished history. The research and scholarship of such leaders in psychotherapy as Jerome Frank, Carl Rogers, and Hans Strupp were central to the establishment of the common-factors approach as viable and important. Rogers (1957) attempted clinically and empirically to tease out the necessary and sufficient factors that lead to therapeutic growth. Personality change for the patient followed from a therapeutic relationship in which the therapist reacted to the patient with accurate empathy, unconditional positive regard, and self-congruence. Frank's (1961) work contained a cross-cultural perspective on healers and psychotherapists and led to the conclusion that the remoralization of a defeated patient and the provision of hope were central to all psychological and moral helping relationships. Strupp and his colleagues (cf. Strupp, Wallach, & Wogan, 1964) pioneered the empirical study of psychodynamic psychotherapy and came to conclusions that were very similar to these findings with regard to the effective ingredients of analytic therapies (Strupp, Hadley, & Gomes-Schwartz, 1977).

Contemporary common-factors investigators have built on these earlier efforts and have been able to demonstrate that most therapies do share a pool of curative ingredients. These common factors are relational and supportive, in that they stem from the therapeutic relationship, and they are technical, in that they derive from the provision of new learning experiences and the opportunities to test new skills in action (Lambert, 1992; Lambert & Bergin, 1994). Each school of psychotherapy probably capitalizes on certain common effective factors and neglects or excludes others. Also, research has demonstrated that certain forms of therapy do have unique effective properties when applied in specific settings to specific populations (Norcross & Newman, 1992). The advantage of this common-factors integration, then, is to increase the number of these curative factors, common and unique, to which the patient may be systematically exposed.

The last type of psychotherapy integration to be considered is theoretical integration. This form of integration has been described as the most sophisticated and important by some writers, but it has been criticized as overly ambitious and essentially impossible by others (Franks, 1984; Lazarus, 1992; Messer, 1992) because of the scientific incompatibilities and philosophical differences among the various schools of psychotherapy. Those who argue in favor of this form of integration do so because of the new perspectives it offers at the levels of theory and of practice. Theoretical integration involves the synthesis of novel models of personality functioning, psychopathology, and psychological change from the concepts of two or more traditional systems. Integrative theories of this kind generally attempt to explain psychological phenomena in interactional terms, by looking for the ways in which environmental, motivational, cognitive, and affective factors influence and are influenced by each other. Causation is usually assumed to be multidirectional and to include conscious and covert factors, and most theoretical integrations include a focus on the ways that individuals re-create past patterns and experiences in the present.

The systems of psychotherapy that follow from such theoretical integration utilize interventions from each of the component theories, as well as lead to original techniques that may "seamlessly blend" two or more therapeutic schools (Wachtel, 1991). At times, the clinical efforts suggested within a theoretically integrated system resemble substantially the choice of techniques of a technically eclectic model. The substantial differences may lie in the belief systems and conceptual explanations that precede the clinical strategies selected by the respective therapists. Theoretical integration goes beyond technical eclecticism in clinical practice by expanding the range of covert and overt factors that can be addressed therapeutically. Subtle interactions between internal states and processes, as well as interactional experiences, can be assessed and targeted for intervention from a number of complementary perspectives. Expected effects of any form of intervention in one or more problem areas can be predicted, tested, and refined as necessary. This conceptual expansion offers a framework in which problems at one level or in one sphere of psychological life can be addressed in formerly incompatible ways (Gold, 1992).

Other types of psychotherapy integration have been proposed and discussed, but these modes have not received much broad attention in the literature. The interested reader is referred to such writers as Schacht (1984), Gold (1992), and Messer (1992) for examples of these integrative forms.

In the next section of this chapter a large number of the major systems of integrative psychotherapy will be introduced and described. They will be grouped in terms of the type of integration that each represents. Of course, it is unlikely that any integrative system will be purely of one type or another, but each is identifiable (by its creator sometimes, and certainly by a reviewer) as fitting most closely into one mode or the other.

THE MAJOR SYSTEMS OF PSYCHOTHERAPY
INTEGRATION

Technical Eclecticism

Eclectic Psychotherapy

Garfield (1980, 1992) has offered eclectic psychotherapy as one of the earliest and most influential versions of a psychotherapy that was based on technical eclecticism. He has emphasized a common-factors approach to the inclusion concepts and methods and has stressed the contributions of the therapeutic relationship in providing support, guidance, hope, and a renewed sense of efficacy. He has also noted that such variables as desensitization and exposure, catharsis, provision of explanations and new information, reinforcement, and training of new skills are the effective ingredients of most influential forms of psychotherapy. Garfield (1992) worked to help the patient utilize these factors by choosing the techniques most often associated with the desired experience, but he was very clear in his belief that the therapeutic interaction is the primary source of change for most patients.

Multimodal Therapy

Multimodal therapy (Lazarus, 1989, 1992) is perhaps the best-known, most widely cited, and most influential version of technical eclecticism in contemporary psychotherapy. Lazarus (1992) was an outspoken critic of attempts at theoretical integration but was equally emphatic about the huge therapeutic advantages offered by a broad-spectrum, eclectic system of assessment and intervention. Multimodal therapy is organized around an extensive assessment of the patient's strengths, excesses, liabilities, and deviant behavior that follows the acronym BASIC ID: Behavior, Affect, Sensation, Imagery, Cognition, Interpersonal relations, and Drugs (or biology). Much attention is paid to the sequential and mutually influential relationships among the covert and behavioral phenomena that are identified as falling into each of these sectors. As the firing order, or casual sequence of variables in the Basic ID, is known, interventions are selected and are implemented. More microscopic Basic ID profiles of discrete or difficult problems and of components of a firing order can be attempted once the initial global assessment and interventions are completed.

Lazarus (1989) stated that he preferred to use methods that have been demonstrated through empirical tests to be effective with specific problems and skill, and his theory and technical strategies are more heavily aligned with social learning theory and with cognitive behavior therapy than with any other therapeutic school. However, his broad-spectrum approach often includes imagery work, techniques drawn from couples and family therapy, gestalt exercises, and some affective and insight-oriented interventions.

Systematic Eclectic Psychotherapy

Systematic eclectic psychotherapy integration is also representative of technical eclecticism and was developed by Beutler and his colleagues (Beutler, 1983; Beutler & Consoli, 1992; Beutler & Hodgson, 1993). Beutler and Hodgson (1993) described this model as a "second-generation" system of integration that attempts to incorporate some of the findings of common-factors theorists into an advanced eclectic approach. This is an empirically informed prescriptive system in which a thorough assessment of the patient is followed by the prescription of the techniques, that have received the most research validation for efficacy with that specific clinical profile, if any such techniques exist. When such research based matching is not possible, techniques are selected according to accumulated clinical findings drawn from the literature and from the experience of the individual therapist. Systematic eclectic psychotherapy therefore resembles multimodal therapy in its general philosophy of eclecticism, as well as in its broad palette of potential interventions. The framework for assessment and for guiding the prescription of interventions is what differentiates this therapy from other eclectic models. Beutler (Beutler & Hodgson, 1993) based the selection of techniques on the interaction of three factors: the stage of psychotherapeutic involvement the patient has reached (drawn from the common-factors literature), the necessary change experiences for which the patient is prepared (based on the studies of Prochaska & DiClemente, 1992a, b) and the dominant aspects of the patient's immediate clinical status and experience. In an assessment of this last factor, a number of components must be included: patient and therapist mediating and long-term goals; the psychological and environmental predisposing factors in the patient's life that are adaptive, pathogenic, and reinforcing of psychopathology; and the condition and affective tone of the therapeutic relationship. Formulation of clinical strategies and techniques is then possible. As necessary and appropriate, interventions can be matched to the ongoing assessment of the patient's needs at four levels: overt dysfunctional behavior, faulty thinking, inhibitions of affective and sensory experience, and repressed unconscious conflict. The choice of intervention is also influenced heavily by the patient's unique coping style, ability to engage in a collaborative therapeutic relationship, and level of reactance or resistance to any type of therapeutic experience. Techniques that can be included in this model range from the interpretive, to exercises that enhance the patient's ability to integrate affect and sensation' to behavioral and cognitive interventions.

Common-Factors Approaches to Psychotherapy Integration

Common-Factors Integration

Beitman's (1992) model of psychotherapy integration, common-factors integration, is an expanded common-factors approach. On an as-needed basis, he added to the overlapping effective ingredients found in the humanistic, existential, cognitive, behavioral, psychodynamic, interpersonal, and systems therapies the useful and specific factors that characterize each. Beitman sought to resolve and correct the faulty self-representations, behavior patterns, and interpersonal cycles that result from unresolved psychological trauma. His therapy is organized around four stages of change: engagement, pattern search, change, and termination. It stresses the combination of enhanced self-observation and of exposure to the feared, avoided sequelae of past trauma as the central mechanisms of change. Techniques may draw from any of the therapies mentioned above. The interventions of the various therapeutic schools lend themselves to the wide variety of self-observation and exposure experiences that are possible in psychotherapy. Specific techniques are selected on the basis of a careful assessment of the unique experiences and changes that may be most helpful to each patient.

Transtheoretical Psychotherapy

Transtheoretical psychotherapy (Prochaska, 1984; Prochaska & DiClemente, 1992a, 1992b) is somewhat difficult to classify as strictly a common-factors or a theoretical type of integrative therapy. As is evident from its name, it is based on a theoretical synthesis, and yet its methods and clinical guidelines are closer to those of the prescriptive models just discussed than to the theoretically integrated models that will be presented below. Transtheoretical therapy guides the therapist in the selection of interventions on the basis of three basic elements of patient assessment: the required change mechanisms, the stage of change at which the patient seeks help, and the level of change that is required. Behavior therapy is indicated in this system for patients who require change at the level of overt symptoms and of maladaptive patterns of dealing with the environment. These interventions are best prescribed when the patient is at the stage of action, which means that the person has a sense of self-liberation and is able to perceive himself or herself as capable of self-control and independent change. The required change mechanisms are those intrinsic in behavioral interventions, including counterconditioning, stimulus control, and contingency management. When the patient requires the change mechanisms of self-reevaluation and self-liberation, suffers from maladaptive cognitions, and is at the stages of contemplation or preparation, then cognitive or rational-emotive therapies are prescribed. The two stages of change mentioned refer to the readiness to examine one's psychological processes and experience, and to be willing to use self-knowledge as a stimulus to change.

Prochaska and DiClemente (1992a) pointed out that interventions aimed at one level or stage of change can and should lead to changes at other levels or stages. For example, the change processes of counterconditioning and stimulus control can be applied to maladaptive cognitions, interpersonal conflicts, or intrapsychic issues, when the patient is at stages of change other than that of action. Mixing of levels, stages, and change mechanisms makes up what are called the *key-level* and *maximum-impact strategies.* In the former, the therapist works in a variety of technical ways to induce change at one level of need that is central in terms of etiology and maintenance. The latter strategy is the use of interventions that impact upon two or more levels in order to create a more substantial and widespread experience of change. However, such efforts are not greatly stressed in this therapy, nor does the theory go very far toward describing the uses and effects of this type of integrative work.

Theoretically Integrated Systems of Psychotherapy

Cyclical Psychodynamics

Perhaps the single most influential system of psychotherapy integration, cyclical psychodynamics, is a theory of personality and of psychotherapy that represents the theoretical integration of concepts and methods drawn from interpersonal psychoanalysis, family systems theory, social learning theory, and behavior therapy (Gold & Wachtel, 1993; Wachtel, 1977; Wachtel & Wachtel, 1986). Cyclical psychodynamic theory is organized around a radically recast view of the causes, role, and meaning of unconscious motives, fantasies, and conflict. This revision suggests that an individual's ongoing social interactions often cause and reinforce unconscious pathogenic processes and anxieties. Thus, unconscious factors in psychopathology may be considered dependent variables that provide information about the patient's current adaptation, perceptions, and relationships. The traditional psychoanalytic view that unconscious issues represent fixations or unresolved desires from one's childhood has been replaced here, though Wachtel (1977) clearly advocated a developmentally oriented understanding of the patient. The effects of the past impinge on the present insofar as the patient's thinking, behavior, and ways of perceiving the self and others have been skewed and deformed through anxiety-engendering interactions with significant others. Cyclical psychodynamics assigns an ironic status to much of a patient's struggle, in that the patient is seen as unintentionally re-creating past internal conflicts and interpersonal binds. As he or she tries to have new experiences, the anxiety-driven warping of perception, thought, and relatedness causes the person to enlist others as "neurotic accomplices" (Wachtel & Wachtel, 1986). Thus, the past is kept alive, ironically, unconsciously and interpersonally, in patterns of dysfunctional behavior, and in correlated internal psychodynamic states.

Integrative psychodynamic therapy (Gold & Wachtel, 1993; Wachtel & McKinney, 1992) is based on this theoretical model and is an open ended amalgam of methods. It is most influenced by psychodynamic, behavioral, and systemic techniques, but it can include any intervention that will interrupt or correct the ongoing, ironic vicious circles in which the patient is caught.

Cognitive-Analytic Therapy

Cognitive-analytic therapy (CAT) is a theoretical integration of psychoanalytic object-relations theory with concepts and clinical methods derived from cognitive therapy (Ryle, 1990; Ryle & Low, 1993). At the level of theory, Ryle demonstrated how conscious planning, decision making, and interpersonal judgment and behavior patterns are structured and determined by unconscious representations of the self in relationship to other internalized persons. Conscious and unconscious functioning and structures of representation are assumed to exist in a mutually influencing and reinforcing relationship. Insofar as a patient is unable to change dysfunctional patterns of thought, behavior, and relatedness, the underlying self and object relationships that prompted these patterns will be confirmed and strengthened as well. These assumptions about the circular nature of pathological processes are central to several of the other integrative systems discussed in this section.

The CAT therapist is concerned primarily with the identification of the ways in which patients fail to learn, specifically, the ways in which patients continue to hold onto their negative assumptions about themselves and the environment. These defective patterns of information processing and of interpersonal engagement resist revision even in the face of new and contrary data. The task of the therapist is to use these object-relational and cognitive formulations to generate explicit descriptions of the patient's "dilemmas," "snags" and "traps": the cycles of negative beliefs, assumptions, fears, enactments, and choices that are self-reinforcing and are driven by overt and unconscious conflict. These descriptions are communicated directly to the patient and become the basis for techniques that are drawn from cognitive and behavior therapy, combined in a sparing way with interpretive work.

Essentially, this is an active instructional therapy in which self-monitoring, cognitive restructuring, and experiential exercises are emphasized to dual ends: to produce changes in symptoms and in thinking, as any traditional cognitive-behavioral therapy would, and to allow new learning to take place so that revisions in the underlying cognitive and object-relational structures can occur as faulty and self-reinforcing cycles are abandoned.

Behavioral Psychotherapy

As developed by Fensterheim (1993), this system is an example of theoretical integration that leads to integrated interventions. Fensterheim (1993) divided the psychological totality of the patient into three levels, Level 1 being the behavioral and Level 3 being the psychodynamic. Level 2 is the level of obstacles and is conceptualized from both the behavioral and the dynamic positions. Its explanatory value lies in formulating the patient's difficulties in working successfully at Level 1. Dynamic conflict, transference and countertransference, and conditioning and reinforcement factors may all be considered here, in isolation or in complex interrelationships.

Fensterheim concentrated most of his assessment efforts at the first, behavioral level, being guided by the law of parsimony, which he cited (1993) as a scientific canon necessitating that if two competing hypotheses are available to explain a phenomenon, the simplest must be preferred. Since behavioral formulations and interventions are much simpler and easier to test than psychodynamic ones, the behavioral level is preferred for both assessment and therapy. Work at the dynamic level proceeds when the patient is not able to make productive use of work at the behavioral level, thus requiring assessment and therapy at Levels 2 and 3. Behavior at Level 1 is examined with regard to the identification of the interpersonal and intrapsychic factors that fueling and maintaining symptoms. When resistances are noted and become too great an interference, other behavioral and dynamic factors are added to the formulation. The dynamic issues of greatest importance in Fensterheim's system are defenses. He noted that, when pathological defenses are made inoperable or are given up, both behavioral change and insight result. Therapy usually proceeds from Levels 1 to 2 and 3 only as necessary. Standard behavioral techniques are often sufficient for instilling changes in the organization of behavior that render the person's defenses obsolete and inoperable. In such cases, change at Levels 2 and 3 occurs spontaneously, as resistances to insight are abandoned and conflicts are resolved.

When straightforward behavioral work is not completely successful, the behavioral measures must be modified and/or complemented by interpretation, in order to deepen and expand the treatment. For example, if it were found during a problematic desensitization procedure that a patient's phobic symptoms were being fueled by an unconscious fear of separation, exposure and extinction of those fears may be worked with through an imagery satiation procedure and through interpersonal exercises, including assertiveness training and relationship enhancement.

Systems-Process Cognitive Therapy

An integration of Bowlby's (1980) attachment theory and cognitive and developmental psychologies makes up the theoretical heart of Guidano's (Guidano, 1987; Guidano & Liotti, 1983) integrative model. He wrote that early disturbances in attachment experiences give rise to tacit or unconscious ways of understanding experience that may dominate the person's behavior and conscious experience in later life. This tacit knowledge is made up of representational or "working models" (Bowlby, 1980) of the self in relation to significant others. The patient's conscious, overt knowledge is linked symbolically to these covert processes and is often unwittingly oriented to the protection or confirmation of these covert assumptions. Additionally, overt knowledge is organized in such a way as to keep the person unaware of, and alienated from, any facets of his or her tacit modes of information processing because of the subjective danger associated with those modes early in life. In persons with psychopathology, tacit knowledge is dominated by assumptions about danger connected with situations that resemble early and failed attachment experiences.

Guidano (1987) noted that two types of change are possible in cognitive therapy. Directive methods, including the standard behavioral and cognitive techniques used in traditional cognitive therapy, result in superficial change: modification of the patient's overt ideas and behaviors without any impact on tacit processes or working models. Deep change occurs only after such surface changes have been made. When the patient becomes less symptomatic and less preoccupied by her or his problems, then memories, emotions, fantasies, dreams, and ideas that are symbolic of covert self- and object representations, or which represent core attachment experiences, will gain access to awareness. The availability of this material in consciousness makes possible a systematic exploration and testing of the basic working models of attachment and of self- and object representation.

The Active Self Model

Another integrative system that exemplifies the approach of theoretical integration is the active self model formulated by Andrews (1990, 1993). This system is organized around a novel theory of personality that places at its center the person's efforts to regulate and to retain a particular self-image. These efforts at homeostasis lead to psychological health if that self-image is flexible, broad, and consistent with the real attributes, strengths, and capacities of the person. Also, healthy functioning is possible to the extent that the maintenance of the self image can be accomplished in the context of productive interpersonal relatedness. Psychological disturbance occurs when the patient's early experiences contribute to any kind of vulnerability and to the formation of a self image that is exaggerated, deviant, or in other ways protective and compensatory. The person who suffers in this way actively structures his or her cognitive, motivational, and affective life — and most significant interactions with others — in ways that are meant to confirm and stabilize the pathological representation of the self. Life becomes a series of dire self fulfilling prophecies. This activity can be carried out in knowing ways, but it is most often unconscious and leads to a growing sense of self-estrangement and to secondary symptoms.

The integrative psychotherapy that is based on the active self theory begins with an assessment of the ways in which the patient engages in negative self-confirmation. Andrews (1993) presented a seven-stage framework for the selection of interventions. Each stage describes the psychological level at which strategies for self-confirmation are manifested: self-concept (Stage 1), motivations (Stage 2a), expectancies and plan (Stage 2b), behavior (Stage 3), others' impressions of the self (Stage 4), others' reactions (Stage 5), selective perceptions of interactions (Stage 6), selective interpretations (Stage 7a), and reactive emotions (Stage 7b). Therapeutic work at all or any relevant stages utilizes interventions from any system that will assist in meeting two goals. The first goal is to increase the patient's awareness of self-confirmatory acts; the second is to help the patient experiment with new ways of being and relating that will lead to a reformulated and more productive self-image. As the self-image changes for the better, the resulting self-confirmatory processes should become more adaptive and should thus promote a new and beneficial feedback cycle at all of the stages.

Process-Experiential Psychotherapy

The process-experiential approach to psychotherapy integration incorporates technical and conceptual aspects from cognitive therapy and Gestalt therapy into a client-centered, experiential-oriented framework (Greenberg, Rice, & Elliot, 1993). This therapy is concerned primarily with highlighting, resolving, and overcoming the blocks to a free moment-to-moment experiencing by the patient. These experiential blockages occur at conscious and unconscious levels and are the expressions of internalized and repetitive criticisms, rebuffs, dangers, and anxieties that have accumulated through interpersonal events. These internal accusers and critics (similar to psychodynamic notions of object representations and cognitive therapy's schemas) manifest themselves in the patient's dysfunctional cognitions, reports of interactions with others, and distortions and inhibitions of emotional life. To allow a gradual revision of concepts of self and other, Greenberg's approach utilizes the foundation of the genuine, accepting, and empathic therapy relationship that is the hallmark of client-centered therapy. He also incorporates active gestalt exercises and methods of cognitive restructuring, which are included to heighten the patient's awareness of experiential blockages and of the processes that interfere with affective and symbolic processing. The patient is then provided with experimental therapeutic situations in which he or she can struggle with, revise, and abandon the psychological structures that limit experiential freedom.

Interpersonal–Cognitive–Experiential Psychotherapy

Another recent and increasingly influential theoretical integration of psychotherapies is Safran's (Reeve, Inck, & Safran, 1993; Safran & Segal, 1990) amalgam of cognitive, interpersonal, and experiential therapies. Safran has viewed the patient's ongoing relationships, in and out of therapy, as the locus of feedback processes that enact, replicate, and reinforce certain pathogenic processes. In particular, the patient "hooks" others into patterns of behavior that confirm ongoing, disturbed interpersonal schemas, which are defined as a "generalized representation of self–other relations" (Reeve, Inck, & Safran, 1993). The collection of interpersonal schemas that are unique to each person reflects and structures the individual's unique view of reality and her or his place and role within that reality. If these interpersonal schemas are more heavily skewed toward grim, dangerous, or difficult scenarios, the person is more likely to develop psychological problems. Troubling interpersonal schemas are manifested clinically by repetitive patterns or interpersonal behavior, through affective disturbances, and by faulty, negative modes of thinking and of processing information. The patient may be more-or-less aware of these interaction cycles and of the cognitive and emotional markers of these problematic ways of functioning.

This theory greatly resembles several of the systems mentioned above, including cyclical psychodynamics, the active self model, and Guidano's integrative position. As in these other models, much of the therapy is aimed at the provision of new experience in and out of therapy. This type of "unhooking" is accomplished through cognitive and experiential techniques. Especially important is therapeutic feedback (metacommunication) about the therapist's experience of the ways in which the patient has attempted to hook him or her into existing maladaptive patterns. These interventions allow the patient to examine more clearly the maladaptive interpersonal cycles and the underlying schemas, and to engage in the process of constructing a new and more adaptive framework for perceiving the self and others.

TOWARD A METAINTEGRATION: THE PLAN OF THIS WORK

Despite important differences in terminology, theoretical foundations, and clinical methods, the integrative models just reviewed (and others not mentioned) have much in common. These systems all rely on the possibility that change will arise through a broad variety of psychology and behavioral events and experiences. Integrative systems admit the fact that no one source of psychotherapeutic improvement exists that is superior to, or more important than, any other. They argue for models of personality that are comprehensive and that acknowledge the importance of all levels of psychological life in pathology and in health: unconscious motivations, conscious experience, affect, cognition, behavior, and interpersonal relationships. They suggest further that each of these realms of experience must be regarded as potentially equivalent to any other as a cause or consequence of abnormal behavior or of health. The idea that change in any single sphere of psychological activity can affect functioning in any other sphere is one that also cuts across the integrative models. The philosophical, theoretical, and clinical barriers that have long kept separate the sectarian therapies are abandoned, although respectfully, and are replaced by a vision of human activity and experience that admits the wisdom of a pluralistic, flexible perspective. Finally, these approaches suggest that human development, adaptation, and psychological growth are far from linear or unidirectional.

In the chapters that follow, the commonalties and convergences among the important integrative efforts are explored in much greater length and depth. Each chapter focuses on one key theoretical or clinical point that is central to psychotherapy in general. The contributions of the psychodynamic, humanistic–experiential, and cognitive–behavioral traditions to our knowledge about these key concepts open each chapter, to be followed by a review of integrative positions. The reviews result in further attempts to synthesize the integrative efforts into a novel, metaintegrative point of view. Finally, the metaintegration is illustrated in an extended case example.

Theories of Personality and Psychopathology

CONTRIBUTIONS OF TRADITIONAL THEORIES TO AN INTEGRATED THEORY OF PERSONALITY AND PSYCHOPATHOLOGY

An integrated theory of personality and of psychopathology must account for the broad range of normal and clinical phenomena that are explained by traditional theories. Further, a novel theory must link advantageously the separate domains and concepts drawn from earlier models. Most important, integrative theories must explain the workings of the normal personality in more inclusive terms than do any of the component systems. Explanations of abnormal behavior must lead to an enhanced understanding of etiology, to the maintenance of ongoing pathology, and, ultimately, to novel, integrative theories and methods of treatment.

In order to consider existing integrative theories we must first turn to the discussion of the relevant contributions to integrative models of personality and of psychopathology made by psychodynamic, humanistic-experiential, and cognitive-behavioral and social learning theories.

Psychoanalysis and its offshoots offer a long and rich tradition of conceptualizing human behavior in terms of motivation, conflict, and defense. All versions of psychodynamic theory stress the unconscious determination of conscious cognition, affect, and behavior, differing predominantly in terms of the particular motives, conflicts, and developmental issues that are viewed as most influential. Classical psychoanalysis posits that personality develops along a path of universal, biologically determined stages of psychosexual wishes. Psychopathology reflects a fixation at, and regression to, unknown and unresolved conflicts stemming from one or more of these fixation points. Symptoms and problem behaviors are understood to reflect several simultaneous covert conflicts, and to be the manifestation of a compromise between the wish to express the unconscious desire and the defensive processes that alter that wish into an unrecognizable form.

Contemporary psychoanalytic theories have retained the emphasis on unconscious motivational factors but have moved toward developmental and etiological models that are more interpersonally and socially conditioned. This conceptual shift within psychoanalysis has been influenced by clinical studies and by the emergence of psychodynamically informed studies of child development (see Mahler, Pine, & Bergman, 1975; Stern, 1985). Collectively, these theories have been described as making up the "relational structure model" (Greenberg & Mitchell, 1983), which emphasizes the interaction between the growing child and the significant persons in his or her life. These interactions are considered crucial in the formation of psychological structures, motivational conflicts, and representations of the self and of others. Relational structure theorists are most concerned with the processes through which the child internalizes, identifies with, and represents productive and maladaptive patterns of relatedness, and with the ways in which these largely unconscious structures skew and distort present-day perception, thinking, affective functioning, and interpersonal engagement.

The relational structure perspective within psychodynamic dynamic thinking refers to any number of separate schools and leading theorists, including self psychology (Kohut, 1977), interpersonal psychoanalysis (Fromm, 1955; Sullivan, 1953), and object relations theory (Greenberg & Mitchell, 1983). The relational structure model that has had the greatest influence on other theorists and therapists, including especially many cognitive-behavioral and integrative writers, has been Bowlby's (1980) representational model of attachment. This theory draws from clinical and research findings and places at its center the child's gradual establishment of prototypes of the self in relation to attachment figures. Psychological health and security result from the internalization of images of parents as reliable and available when the child is in need of comfort, protection, or encouragement for exploration. Psychological disturbance is the outcome of troubled experiences around attachment and separation in childhood that form the basis for repetitive cognitive structures and patterns of information processing in the adult that provoke anxiety, insecurity, self-doubt, and other precursors of pathology. Attachment theory is very similar to the other versions of relationally oriented psychodynamic models in these ways and also bears a striking resemblance, as we will see below, to theories of personality that are based on cognitive schemas.

The individual theories and theorists included in the group of humanistic and experiential therapists often differ considerably with regard to the specifics and fine points of personality and psychopathology. However, on the whole, client-centered theories (Raskin & Rogers, 1989; Rogers, 1957), Gestalt theory (Perls, 1973), and existential theories (Bugental & Kleiner, 1993; May, 1977; Yalom, 1981) demonstrate substantial agreement about the core issues of psychological health and disturbance (Rice & Greenberg, 1992).

Humanistic and experiential theories share a concern with human potential and with the ways in which psychological growth, authenticity, and integration can be achieved or are thwarted. Realization and integration of the person's abilities, values, and goals; emotional and cognitive flexibility and openness; a capacity for genuine self-acceptance; and warm, empathic regard for others — these are some of the signs of self-actualization that are mentioned in the literature (e.g., Maslow, 1954; Rogers, 1961). Humanistic theorists generally adopt a phenomenological orientation to the study of other persons (Rice & Greenberg, 1992). Their chief empirical and clinical concerns are the ongoing states of experience and awareness that reflect moments either of authentic living, or of unhealthy and avoidant functioning. Each theory in this group stresses one or more aspects of experience and phenomenology. Gestalt therapy is most concerned with the person's openness to the processes of moment-to-moment bodily, cognitive, and emotional experience (Perls, Goodman, & Hefferline, 1951). Rogers (1961) and other client-centered therapists (Gendlin, 1984; Levant & Shlein, 1984; Raskin & Rogers, 1989; Rice, 1984) emphasize the ability to consciously symbolize what one is experiencing as a critical factor in the process of self-actualization. Existential writers agree with the criterion of unimpeded awareness but are more concerned with the individual's capacity to stay with and to face fully life's painful existential realities.

Humanistic theories are teleological in their emphasis on the role of the person's perceptions of the future in shaping the experience of the present. These tend to deemphasize developmental models and the role of past experience. Similarly, most writers in this tradition have attempted to focus explicitly on issues of individual free will and choice in behavior and adaptation (Bugenthal & Kleiner, 1993; May & Yalom, 1989). Behavioral and psychodynamic models are criticized by many in this group as overly deterministic and historical. Such concepts, humanistic therapists often argue, deny the active participation of the person in his or her life. Deterministic theories tend to portray the person as passive and often overlook the constructive and forward-looking trends that may be present in latent forms, even in the most disturbed person.

Psychopathology is thought to result from chronic anxiety or other threats that become associated with any particular experiences, emotions, or thoughts of the self and others. Any event or inner state that is associated with some subjective danger to the person may thus eventuate in a closing down, interruption, or distortion of awareness. The person is diverted from the process of self-actualization. Instead, he or she engages in mechanized, rigid, and inauthentic interactions within the self and with others. Spontaneous experiencing, a process that is based on the ability to symbolize psychological phenomena completely and immediately, is replaced by controlled, dulled, or exaggerated inner states and behaviors. These temporarily comforting alterations of the ability to be aware and to live fully help the person to avoid internal distress, but lead to a profound sense of alienation from the self and from others.

Different schools of thought in this group have formulated competing, yet not incompatible, concepts of the etiology of anxiety and alienation from the self. Existential therapists (Bugenthal & Kleiner, 1993; May, 1977; Yalom, 1981) have suggested that anxiety is an inevitable consequence of human existence. The "thrown," helpless nature of the person in the face of life's inevitable limits (including freedom, meaninglessness, finitude, isolation, separation, and death) yields a sense of uncertainty and insecurity that is part of the experience of each of us (Bugenthal & Kleiner, 1993). To the degree that the person is unable or unwilling to acknowledge these issues and anxieties, his or her experience and way of life will be guided by the goal of avoidance and escape. When such goals become predominant and pervasive, psychic disturbance results.

Client-centered and Gestalt therapists probably would not disagree with these last ideas, but they would also stress the role of learning and of interpersonal interaction in the etiology of psychopathology. Anxiety is seen by client-centered therapists (Rice & Greenberg, 1992; Rogers, 1959) as resulting from a conflict between the need to preserve a learned image of the self and any experience that is incompatible with that image. Learned self-images (the "ideal self" referred to by Rogers, 1959) result from repeated evaluations of the person by parents and other significant persons during childhood. To the degree that important constructive experiences are disapproved of by these authorities (e.g., the need to express disappointment in one's parents), those tendencies will mean danger to that person in the future. Gaining the approval of others supersedes actualization of the self as an aim at those moments. Further, those experiences will be excluded from the ideal self-image the person constructs, so that any awareness of such trends will lead to incongruity, anxiety, and limitations of awareness. Gestalt therapy (Perls, 1973) broadly concurs with this etiological model, suggesting that anxiety and experiential limits accrue from the internalization of interpersonal and societal sanctions on certain types of experience.

The earliest work in behavior therapy was based on mainstream versions of learning theory that stressed the ways in which maladaptive habits, behavior patterns, and symptoms are acquired through the processes of classical and operant conditioning (see Salter, 1949; Wolpe, 1958). Behavior therapists in those beginning years were concerned exclusively with overt behaviors and scorned the "mentalism" and lack of empirical validity that they attributed to traditional theories of personality (Eysenck, 1960). Of course, there were a few important exceptions to this exclusively behavioral position. In the academic world, theorists such as Hull (1952) developed laboratory-based learning theories that included organismic or cognitive constructs as mediating processes. Clinicians such as Mowrer (1953) also produced conditioning- and reinforcement-based theories that took seriously the role of covert processes in determining behavior and psychopathology.

As academic psychology became more oriented to the "cognitive revolution," behaviorally oriented personality theorists and clinicians began to include cognitive and perceptual processes in their models in more explicit and central ways. The learning processes that were emphasized were expanded beyond the limits of the Pavlovian and Skinnerian models to one that placed the acquisition of behavior solidly in the context of social and interpersonal interactions (Bandura & Walters, 1963; Bowers, 1973; Mischel, 1973). Social learning theorists accepted the power of learning through classical and operant conditioning but also stressed the importance of observational learning, modeling of social behavior, and identification with peers and with authorities. These authors also reported on the impressive role

of the person's subjective organization of, and expectancies about, the
social context in the determination of behavior.

In the 1980s and 1990s, social learning and behavioral theories
models have yielded to a great degree to even more cognitively dominated models of learning and personality (Stein & Young, 1992). This
movement reflects a general trend within academic psychology and
in psychotherapy toward subjectively oriented, cognitive process
models and theories (Gold, 1995). These advances have placed the
modes and structures of representing and organizing experience at
the center of understanding of both normal and abnormal phenomena.
Somewhat amazingly, certain cognitive and behaviorally oriented
theorists have begun to take seriously the notion of unconscious processing and its central role in psychopathology (Mahoney, 1991). Others in this group have worked out comprehensive theories of
personality and psychopathology that are quite similar to the work
of Bowlby (1980) and other dynamic relational structure theorists (see
above). This new wave of cognitive theorists includes such writers
as Bandura (1977), who advanced the notion of an interpersonally
derived, cognitively represented self. Bandura suggested that the goal
of much of the person's activity is focused on gaining and maintaining
the experience and perception of the self as effective. Beck, Freeman,
and Associates (1989), Young (1992), and others, acknowledging a
debt to pioneers such as Piaget (1926) and Kelly (1955), have presented personality theories in which the central concept is the
schema. Schemas are defined as the broad conceptual prototypes that
organize specific experiences. They operate at all levels of awareness
and give rise to conscious thoughts, feelings, and behaviors.

Thus, the specifics of any cognitive-behavioral understanding of
psychopathology depend on the point at which the individual writer
is located on the theoretical continuum described above. Traditional
learning-theory-based approaches (e.g., Wolpe, 1958) regarded abnormal processes as being derived from failed or skewed patterns of conditioning, reinforcement, and generalization. Expanded models of
behavior therapy, like that of Goldfried and Davison (1976, 1994),
retain these explanatory concepts but add to them by acknowledging
the importance of observational learning and faulty cognition in the
acquisition of symptoms and abnormal behaviors. In these latter models, there is an emphasis on dysfunctions of self-talk, planning, self-
control, and decision making, and it is assumed that behavior and
cognition exist in a mutually influential relationship.

Cognitive theorists, particularly Beck (1976), rely on all of the
learning concepts mentioned above to explain the etiology of distur-

bance, but they stress conflict and trauma in interpersonal relationships as the source of pathogenic cognitive structures and contents. Cognitive therapists are most concerned with the role of conscious thinking and of underlying schemas in the acute production and chronic maintenance of disturbance. Ellis (1984) was equally emphatic about the centrality of irrational beliefs and schemas in pathology but argued that these ways of thinking are biologically and genetically determined. Regardless of their theories of etiology, all cognitive theorists stress the determining effects of dysfunctional beliefs on behavior, affect, and patterns of interpersonal relatedness. However, these variables are seen as existing in a reinforcing feedback loop with the antecedent cognitions. Disturbed interactions and emotions perpetuate the thoughts and structures that elicited them.

INTEGRATIVE THEORIES OF PERSONALITY AND PSYCHOPATHOLOGY

Integrative theories of personality tend to reflect and build on the convergences in the sectarian schools that were just described. The syntheses of psychodynamic, humanistic, and social learning approaches that have been achieved are highly similar to each other, and to some of the more contemporary versions of the original theories.

At the core of most integrative theories are developmental, cognitive, and epistemological concepts that are congenial to many contemporary psychoanalysts, cognitive behaviorists, and experiential theorists. The perceptual and information-processing activity of people in constructing representational models of themselves in action with others is crucial and almost universal across current thinking about personality (Neimeyer, 1993; Neimeyer & Feixas, 1990). It seems to matter little, if at all, whether these ways of knowing and structures of representation are called cognitive styles (Shapiro, 1965), self or interpersonal schemas (Guidano, 1987, 1991; Horowitz, 1988; Reeve et al., 1993), self and object representations (Gold, 1990a, b; Ryle, 1990; Wachtel, 1985), or working models (Bowlby, 1980). These labels appear to differ semantically, with subtle differences that are unimportant when the concepts are applied carefully. As Weston (1988) pointed out, there is considerable overlap among the many theoretical approaches to the concepts of self and perception of others and the ways in which people construct models of reality and construe and permanently represent themselves and their interactions with others. What is important in these discussions is the heavy weight accorded to the personal modes of knowing in which images at self and of others are embedded. These cognitive processes and structures are the basic framework of character or personality (Barnett, 1980; Holt, 1989).

A social learning perspective in which real interactions are the basic developmental stuff of intrapsychic representational structure is a shared piece of the integrative approach. Attachment theory is one model of representational development that organizes many integrative theories of personality (e.g., Gold & Stricker, 1993; Guidano, 1987; Safran & Segal, 1990). Other integrative theorists such as Wachtel (1977; Gold & Wachtel, 1993) find guidance in interpersonal developmental models drawn from the work of Horney (1950) and Sullivan (1953), or from psychoanalytic object relations theories (Allen, 1993; Horowitz, 1988; Ryle, 1990). Again, regardless of the specific theory of development accepted by any writer, there is substantial convergence with regard to the processes of learning and internalization. Social learning gives rise to the internal structures that are prototypes for the ongoing organization of experience. These internalized remnants of early life are the building blocks of the adult's self-images, perceptions of others, motives, fears, affects, and morality.

Behavior, cognition, affect, interpersonal scripts, and character are formed in the slow process of social maturation. Ongoing experience is remembered both in the narrow sense of memory and in the broader form of representational modes of knowing. Integrative theories stress that the person's representational models are linked to overt behavior in a complex system of feed forward and feedback loops. Covert experiential models inform the person about his or her place in the world and generate internal scripts for human interaction that come to guide much of behavior. These scripts (see Guidano, 1991; Horowitz, 1988) may be covert or conscious and are extremely influential with regard to the irony of psychopathology and the generation of anxiety and other psychological discomforts. A pathogenic script expresses the person's unwitting construction of an intrapsychic or interpersonal experience as subjectively threatening. The images and actions that are prescribed by that script are meant to lead to a different and more positively toned outcome than the original experiences that are "remembered" in the representational structures. However, as will be discussed below, because of the limits placed on the person's choices, ironic repetition often prevails. It is in the representational sphere of psychological life that integrative efforts usually include the premise of unconscious mental activity. People tend to be unaware of their ways of constructing experience, and especially when pathology is present, dynamic reasons exist for remaining unaware of central, anxiety-laden images of the self and of others. Affectively oriented information processing, ongoing appraisal of the self and of others, and efforts to maintain a sense of identity and homeostasis are among the acknowledged unconscious operations that figure prominently in behavior and experience (Guidano & Liotti, 1983; Ryle, 1990; Safran & Segal, 1990).

Unlike most psychoanalytic theories (with the exception of those of such mavericks as Alexander & French, 1946, or Horney, 1950), integrative models of unconscious activity suggest that these variables exist in an open, cyclical relationship with ongoing behavior and cognition, as described above. Consideration of defense mechanisms is not restricted to the intrapsychic activities, such as repression or denial (A. Freud, 1936), that are the focus of psychoanalysis, though such processes are of great importance in integrative models. Instead, any aspect of behavior or mental activity can be seen to play a part in the avoidance of inner states or of being aware of some domain of interpersonal experience (Fensterheim, 1993).

Integrative theories share a cyclical, process-oriented perspective on the problem of causality in which all levels of experience and psychology are understood to be relevant and interrelated. This means that unconscious motives, conscious cognition, experience, and emotions, overt behavior, and interpersonal input are all seen as potential sources of activity and experience. Rather than search for first causes or engage in rigid definitions of cause-and-effect relationships in an a priori manner, integrative theories seek to portray the multidirectional relationships that exist among all of these factors (Gold, 1992). Circular models of personality avoid the problem of reductionism in that no one aspect of behavior need be considered superficial, redundant, or epiphenomenal. Similarly, the division between nature and nurture, or between trait and environmental theories, is avoided. Biology, intrapsychic factors, and context are understood to influence each other inevitably, and to be inseparable with regard to concerns about which variable came first. Psychic structure, motivation, and conflict are considered dependent on interpersonal reinforcement by current relationships, as well as by covert intrapersonal processes (Ryle, 1990; Safran & Segal, 1990; Fensterheim, 1993, Gold & Wachtel, 1993; Wachtel, 1977). The normal personality is considered an open system that is flexible and yet is continuous over time. Subjective states such as a stable identity, which grows and changes slowly throughout one's life, are the phenomenological manifestation of this underlying structure. Of critical importance clinically is the extent to which the person's construction of reality allows for open, confident construal of the self and the world. Psychopathological functioning represents some interference in the personality system. Such interruptions may be found either in the closing of the person to new experience and change or in a lack of stability and continuity within the personality over time. Such interference is usually viewed as reflecting a representational system that is dominated by schemas that cause the person to perceive herself or himself as vulnerable in some important way. The perception of vulnerability causes the person to sacrifice openness to avoidant modes of construing the world, thereby transforming a growth-oriented system into one that is self-contained and is marked by repetition.

Integrative views of personality are marked by a vision of human beings as active agents, who are engaged in the construction, representation, and interpretation of their environment and experiences. These theories reflect a discomfort with the extreme determinism that typifies both classical psychoanalysis and radical versions of behaviorism. However, most integrative positions also fall short of endorsing and incorporating the actualizing, teleological, and freewill perspectives of humanism and existentialism. Instead, integrative theories suggest that human behavior is determined in part by prior learning, by biological limits, and particularly by the cognitive, emotional, and characterological skewings that result from past interpersonal experience. At the same time, these theories suggest that there exist within the person tendencies to overcome the past, to reconstruct representations of the self and of others, and to indeed live authentically and fully. The healthy person is able to learn from new experiences, to use old knowledge and experience in a flexible, problem-solving way, and to continually revise and modify thought, perceptions, and images of the self and of others. Free access to spontaneous emotion, to imagination, and to bodily sensation are also part of the makeup of psychological health. This potential for active revision of the self, of patterns of construing experience, and of regulating interaction with others in a positive direction is implicitly a part of most major integrative theories. For example, in Andrew's (1993) active self theory, the person who is free of the need to reinforce certain defensive, compensatory self-images can engage in a wide range of intrapsychic and interpersonal experiences. This broad palette of events will produce for that person new information, affects, and interactions that will lead to intrapsychic change in the form of the expansion of the self-representation, and to personal growth. Cyclical psychodynamic theory (Wachtel, 1977) and versions of integrative theory that derive from cognitive, attachment, and interpersonal theories (Guidano, 1988; Ryle, 1990; Safran & Segal, 1990) share the implicit assumption that psychological health is marked by the gradual assimilation of new experiences into existing psychological structures and processes, to be followed by revisions in those internal guides.

The manifestations of psychopathology are found in any and all domains of behavior and experience. The unique contribution of integrative approaches does not lie in this recognition, which is shared by virtually all students of abnormal psychology. Instead, integrative theories advance our knowledge by offering a model that gives equal importance to the behavioral, interpersonal, cognitive, experiential, psychodynamic, and structural features and contributions to psychological disturbance. Such a perspective does not require reduction or translation of one set of phenomena into another, theoretically more desirable set of issues. Any process in any domain of experience may be clinically significant on its own. Strict assumptions about causal relationships between psychic domains are subordinated to a systemic clinical observation.

Considerable agreement exists among integrationists that disturbances of personality are caused chiefly by anxiety (Beier, 1966; Feather & Rhoades, 1972a; Ryle, 1990; Safran & Segal, 1990; Wachtel, 1977; Fensterheim, 1993; and many others). Anxiety is typically considered a socially learned response to any internal state, thought, behavior, or interpersonal situation that is experienced and represented by the person as threatening or dangerous. There are many possible familial and social precursors to such destructive constructions of reality. Anxiety and psychopathology are derived from any interactions with parents and other important adults that convince the growing child of his or her vulnerability to loss, attack, guilt, shame, unworthiness, or deficiency.

High levels of anxiety limit the person's ability to learn (Sullivan, 1953) and close the personality system to new influences. As a result, preexisting patterns of responding become dominant, chiefly those that were most successful in eliminating or managing anxiety.

Symptoms of psychopathology are embedded in the person's current way of life, which is dominated by unwitting and unintended replication of the past failures, pain, or traumas that were the historical sources of the current anxiety (Fensterheim, 1993; Linehan, 1993; Ryle, 1990; Safran & Segal, 1990; Wachtel, 1977). Avoidant functioning that is based on prior learning, experience, and internalization may lead to any combination of the following: behavioral excesses or deficits; interpersonal failure, frustration, or conflict; gaps in social skills, problem solving, and intellectual achievement; cognitive distortions, deficits, and exaggerations; inhibitions or amplifications of experience, affect, anxiety, and sensation; and unconscious motivational and moral conflicts. Most integrative writers opt for a position regarding the relationships between these variables that is divorced from traditional, directional models of determinism. Wachtel (1977, 1993; Gold & Wachtel, 1993) suggested that an "ironic" vision of psychopathology is more descriptive of human activity and agency than is the internally deterministic "tragic" vision contained within psychoanalysis, cognitive-behavioral therapy's environmentally "comic" vision, or humanistic psychology's "romantic vision" of unfolding and blocked potentials (Messer, 1992).

The ironic vision on which integrative theories rest posits that people unknowingly recreate old fears, relationships, and conflictual experiences while intending to do otherwise. In particular, the troubled person's attempts to surmount and change his or her old patterns, connections, and conflicts repeatedly take him or her back to the same undesirable points (Gold & Wachtel, 1993). These undesired and unanticipated consequences result from biased, faulty ways of constructing experience and from skill deficits that arose when earlier learning was interrupted. Anxiety-provoking experiences that subjectively threaten the person's sense of psychological well-being and equilibrium are critical factors that lead to a reduced capacity to benefit from new learning and to revise internal structures and meanings. With this limited ability to shake off the effects of past meanings and events, the person cannot help but re-create the past again and again.

Other integrative theories that stress the agency of the self (Andrews, 1993; Guidano, 1987; Ryle & Low, 1993; Safran & Segal, 1990) are marked by this ironic perspective. They all recognize the self as operating actively, in a search for novel experiences and meanings, and yet as limited by anxiety that is derived from internal representations of former events. Thus, ongoing experience is colored unavoidably by the tension between the person's desires and efforts to modify, on the one hand, and to preserve, on the other, old behavior patterns, interpersonal interactions, and modes of perceiving the self and of finding and encoding meaning and affects. To the degree that the need for security, stability, and sameness wins out over the desire for change, ironic consequences may dominate the person's existence.

Past experience and unresolved conflict are essential variables in any integrative theory of psychopathology; yet these issues are understood in unique ways. Wachtel (1977) has argued cogently against the "frozen" existence of childhood drives, defenses, and fixations. He substituted for this "woolly mammoth" metaphor a process orientation to the past. The past remains alive and powerful as a result of the present. The past exists in and influences the present, insofar as ways of representing experience, of thinking, and of behaving remain relatively unchanged as the person ages. Conflicts, motives, and fears that seem to be remnants of childhood may actually be dependent variables; that is, ironic products of present-day functioning (Gold & Wachtel, 1993; Wachtel, 1977, 1993). The central importance of ongoing behavior, relationships, and experience in keeping alive early schematic, affective, and motivational structures and issues is a shared emphasis across virtually all of the explicit and intrinsic integrative theories. The critical reinforcing events in this cycle are repetitive, maladaptive, and defensive interactions within the self and with others (Fensterheim, 1993; Ryle & Low, 1993). These result in the confirmation of previously acquired pathogenic self-images (Andrews, 1993), the reinforcement of old maladaptive interpersonal schemas (Reeve et al., 1993), and the continuation of apparently regressive unconscious fantasies and conflicts (Wachtel, 1993).

A METATHEORY OF PERSONALITY AND PSYCHOPATHOLOGY: THE ORGANIZING ROLE OF PERSONAL NARRATIVES

Any advance in theorizing about personality and psychopathology must be able to account for human behavior in more comprehensively than did preceding efforts. Collectively, the integrative models discussed above represent a major advance. Integrative theories offer a process orientation that recognizes the importance of all levels of experience, one in which all psychological domains of human activity are included as influential in their own right. Perhaps the most important contribution of these approaches is the focus on the circularity of both healthy and abnormal behavior. The contextual and multidirectional view of causation and of the maintenance of disturbance acknowledges and transcends the contributions and traditions of the dynamic, humanistic, and social learning models.

However, implicit in these advances are certain shortcomings and limitations that need to be addressed. In the zeal to advance a process approach, integrative theories seem to lose some of the richness of experiential content that marks the sectarian theories. One result is a leveling of impact on and within the individual of all potential causative factors, be they motivational, cognitive, affect, or environmental. Yet most clinicians would agree that, for many individuals, reinforcement from without is critical and exclusively potent, and that to many others the tragic vision of psychoanalytic unconscious determinism is most applicable. Similarly, the circular, ironic vision of causality contained in most integrative work is crucially important yet does not always match the seemingly fixed and historically regressive clinical presentation of many patients. The drama, passion, and irrational nature of much of human experience, particularly of abnormal functioning, seem at times to be partially absent from integrative models.

Existing integrative models also do not address fully the role and place of the broad political, historical, and sociocultural system in which the individual lives. Only a very few integrative contributions have included a discussion of these factors, and of the ethnic, sexual, economic, moral, and ideological issues that shape each person (Cushman, 1995; Gold, 1992; Healey, 1993; Rubin, 1993; Wachtel, 1989). As a result, these contextual integrative theories of personality and psychopathology are paradoxically situated in somewhat anonymous terms with regard to the broader context in which people actually live.

How, then, may the best of the new integrative theories be expanded and elaborated to preserve both the richness of their predecessors and their own creative additions? One possibility, which will be returned to throughout the remainder of this book, is the use of the concept of *narrative* as a theoretical framework that subsumes other conceptual systems. Narrative, story-telling, or the thematic organization of experience has recently emerged as a central organizing variable in cognitive psychology (Oatley, 1992), personality psychology (Berzonsky, 1993; Herman, 1993), folk psychology, and developmental psychology (Bruner, 1990), as well as many forms of psychotherapy (Cushman, 1995; Lyddon, 1992; Schafer, 1976; Spence, 1982; White & Epson, 1990). It may also serve as a conceptual framework for integrating psychotherapies and the theories on which they are based.

Narratives are the stories of each person's life and experience. Narration is the process of constructing and retaining meaning out of the rich raw data of experience (Bruner, 1990). Thus, the use of this construct allows the incorporation in an immediate and experientially near fashion of the emphasis on representational structures and processes that is found in integrative models. Narratives are also infinitely rich in content, thus addressing the advantages of traditional theories and of integrative models. They exist both within and outside of awareness, and provide the person with a structure for interpreting, representing, and recording his or her impressions of the self and of interpersonal and environmental events.

A narrative does not exist in a physical sense. It is an inferred construct that allows the observer, and perhaps eventually the person, to thematically understand and organize the direction of a person's life. Narratives subsume and structure the traditional variables that are included in traditional and integrative personality theories. Any individual's life story contains some reference to motivation, intrapersonal and interpersonal consistency and conflict, a plot, and an environmental setting with other actors, sociocultural institutions, and group events. The plot in the narrative contains the thoughts, emotions, bodily experiences, memories, ideologies, verbalizations, and overt behaviors of the narrator, and of the significant people and groups in the narrator's life. The person may be aware completely of all, many, some, or few of these narrative components and may in fact have developed subsidiary stories (the defense mechanisms of psychoanalysis or the symbolic failures of humanistic theories) that confirm, avoid, or distort the central thematic issues of the major narrative strand. Narratives also contain some remnants of past experience, a construction and description of the person's current life situation, and references to, and anticipation of, the future.

A narrative resembles, and may entirely overlap with, the schematic representational structures posited in personality theories; yet a narrative is also closer to and is part of immediate awareness. Narrative representations are dynamic and are not separated from the affective, motivational, and social spheres of action. Thinking, feeling, perception, and behavior are guided by one's personal story, and in turn, these activities exist in the reinforcing, confirming relationship described in many integrative theories.

It is likely that each individual has several important narratives, or components of narratives, that exist in a complementary or conflicting pattern of influence. Herman (1993) described the working of personality as that of a polyphonic model. To extend his metaphor, the polyphony may be known to the person or may blend into a blur, to be heard only by the outsider. Some of the alternative voices may be known to the person, while others may operate outside of awareness. The person, then, can have multiple, contradictory, and competing self-images that reflect several narratives or stories about the self. He or she holds onto parallel, multiple object representations that are based on narratives about others, and on any number of plots, plans, or scripts (stories about how to be, what to think, feel, and do in the presence of certain persons, social tasks, or cultural, social, or ideological challenges).

The historical "truth" of individual narratives is currently the subject of much discussion in the philosophical, psychological, and psychotherapeutic literature (Cushman, 1995; Greenberg et al., 1993; Spence, 1982; White & Epson, 1990). If a consensus of opinion does exist at this point, it is one arguing that personal narratives represent the individual's best effort at constructing meaning: making sense of, and being able to tell himself or herself about, what has happened, who he or she is, and where her or his life is going. In this view, narratives are fictional or made up, yet are subjectively true. They are composed of the stuff of experience as filtered and interpreted through the idiosyncratic cognitive, affective, and moral matrix that each person possesses. Narrative theories are a specific version of constructivist thinking and are part of the general domain of the specialty of hermeneutics (Cushman, 1995; Gill, 1994; Greenberg et al., 1993). These disciplines are concerned primarily with the ways in which each of us finds and creates meaning from the mass of sensation, data, and action to which we are constantly exposed.

A productive narrative is oriented toward future possibilities and goals. In it, the person portrays herself or himself as effective, lovable, and worthy of success and satisfaction. Self-descriptions overlap with the impressions and reactions of others in terms of the person's abilities and capacities. Within reasonable limits, other people are seen as available, reliable, and valuable, and the world is described as manageable, safe, predictable, and attractive. The story includes significant space for internal and interpersonal conflict, but these experiences are viewed as resolvable and as leading to growth. The structure and content of the narrative encourage full access to motives, feelings, thoughts, and a wide range of actions, as these factors are parts of positive story lines. The past is referred to for guidance and enrichment but is not a source of preoccupation.

Narratives place the person inside or outside some broader social, political, economic, and ideological context. Each person's story lines omit or contain these macroscopic variables in an idiosyncratic and highly important amalgam. These cultural aspects of the story about the self in the world interact with other themes and subplots in neutral, positive, or negative ways. In a productive narrative, the person construes the larger world as providing opportunities, as a place where he or she belongs and is accepted, and as a reasonably inviting and provisioned setting. The disturbed person may envision herself or himself as alienated, rebellious, persecuted, or in other ways deprived and isolated by an unfair, hostile, and meaningless society.

The productive narrative allows the process of self-actualization to proceed to the most complete degree that is possible. Since the person's story does not prohibit or shun any aspects of experience, avoidance of self or of others need not occur. As a result, new learning can take place, and as new information and experience is assimilated, the structure and content of the narrative change. It may be this process that accounts for the interplay of a stable yet evolving identity with changing life events.

The narratives that are implicated in psychological dysfunctions may be described as "broken," distorted, fragmentary, or inappropriate to the person's immediate and sociocultural circumstances. Narrative difficulties may occur consciously or unwittingly at any or all levels of psychological life: social, behavioral, moral, cognitive, experiential, and motivational. Pathology inducing narratives are organized around a portrayal of a self that has lost control of life, and that is vulnerable, despised, impaired, or distorted in some other major way. These stories are derived from the individual's interpretation of accumulated interpersonal experience. They may or may not reflect accurately the "true" characteristics of the person or of the feelings and attitudes of others. The story lines that evolve from such a self-portrayal tend to aim at obtaining a sense of security and safety at the cost of the person's individuality, autonomy, basic needs, and goals. Such plots involve efforts to hide one's weaknesses from himself or herself and from others or to go after compensation or revenge for previous suffering.

Any of the elements of a narrative may be highlighted, exaggerated, left out, or distorted in the service of, or as a result of, such defensive efforts. This process is reminiscent of Andrews' (1993) descriptions of self-confirmatory processes, or of the vicious circles described by Safran and Segal (1990), Ryle (1990), Wachtel (1993), and many others. Quite often, pathogenic narratives have the ironic consequences described by these integrative writers. The problematic, excessive, or deficient cognitions, affects, interpersonal patterns, and unconscious conflicts that are generated by disturbed stories frequently lead people to experiences that reinforce and maintain their fears and impressions of themselves and of the world. However, many patients present with narratives that are better described as tragic or comedic. In the former, the intrapsychic aspects of behavior that are unformulated in the narrative (unconscious conflict, unsymbolized experience, and representational deficits or distortions) exert a deterministic influence on the person. This type of pathology may not depend on external vicious circles. In fact, such narratives may seem to override any environmental input. Tragic and poorly articulated narratives decrease the person's sensitivity to the interpersonal world by creating preoccupations with inner states and structures of which the person paradoxically remains unaware. In the end, ongoing relationships within the person are the maintaining factors in the narrative.

Patients with an overwhelmingly comedic narrative portray and experience themselves as helpless in the face of external events and forces, and such a narrative may in fact lead to the realization of this type of situation. For these patients, intrapsychic factors and ironic vicious circles may also play a diminished role in certain or many aspects of psychopathology.

It is likely that most problematic narratives contain elements of tragedy, irony, comedy, and romance. Therefore, each patient will bring to therapy his or her unique blend of unconsciously determined, interactional, and environmentally contingent disturbances. Certain disturbing narratives cause the patient to function as if he or she were stuck in the past, causing a subjective sense (both for the person and for the observer) of fixation or regression to earlier levels of development. These narratives are structured around a self-portrayal of the person as more childlike, helpless, or subordinate than he or she may be in actuality. This type of story about the self is linked to plots in which other people are seen as more adultlike, stronger, and more capable. In this scenario, new skills cannot be integrated because no internal framework exists for observation, learning, and practice. The end results are cognitive, affective, and social deficits that confirm and maintain the past as the temporal location of the person's life. Present and future are barely acknowledged and, when they are, only as pale shadows of what has already been told and known. Such ongoing re-creation of the past may occur in narratives that lean toward the tragic, comedic, or ironic. The specific ways in which the person sees the past as ongoing are shaped by the type of vision in which he or she lives.

CLINICAL APPLICATION OF THE
METATHEORETICAL MODEL

The integrative therapist shifts from one vision to the other as clinical needs dictate, without having to abandon or to overemphasis any. The therapist examines and makes explicit, in cooperation with the patient, the broad outline and direction of the patient's guiding narrative. As the details, subplots, themes, history, and characters are filled in, therapist and patient begin to work together with this raw material. It is perused for signs of gaps and for underlying motivations that are influential but that remain unsymbolized or only dimly perceptible. The distortions of experience that represent conflict, defenses, and underlying representational structures are noted as well. Emotional and experiential themes, exaggerations, and difficulties are acknowledged and explored, as are the thoughts, behaviors, images, and physical sensations that make up the moment-to-moment stuff of the narrative. The cast of the characters who were formative in this narrative are the subject of much inquiry, as are the current figures who are described as the major persons in the patient's life. Omissions of significant others, or devalued, idealized, or distorted descriptions of interactions, are very important. The various portrayals of the self and the ways in which the person finds or avoids pleasure, pain, meaning, and purpose are of course central to the investigation of the narrative. All of these issues may sometimes be easily known by the patient, but often, the elements of the narrative are out of awareness and must be interpreted and inferred. This is particularly the case with conflictual, painful scripts, plots, and stories about the self in relation to past and present relationships that are emotionally crucial to the patient.

Most narratives contain elements of the ironic, tragic, comedic, and romantic visions, though each individual story line will probably be dominated by one or two of these perspectives. Clinically, once the narrative is understood to some degree, its contribution to the patient's pathology is formulated, sometimes silently and exclusively by the therapist as an internal guide to intervention, and sometimes as an explicit, shared framework for collaboration.

In the remainder of this chapter, the case of James is used as an example of the formulation and clinical use of an integrated narrative structure. James is discussed in each subsequent chapter as well, and his narrative is used to illustrate clinically the integrative concepts around which all of the following chapters of this book are based.

James was a middle-class, married Caucasian in his mid-30s who sought psychotherapy because of long-standing work-related difficulties. He was a technical writer for a large electronics company who wrote and edited the company newsletter, press releases and publicity statements, and consumer manuals for home entertainment products. His work was excruciatingly difficult because of deadline pressures that he found almost impossible to meet because of his perfectionism, obsessive concern with accuracy and detail, and inability to feel certain that he had completed a task satisfactorily and completely. He would stop the presses over and over again to check his work and to change the slightest and most insignificant details, and he felt totally preoccupied with this process. He reported that he feared humiliation at the hands of his superiors for his incompetence, and he expected to be fired at any moment. These fears and images persisted despite repeated reassurances by his superiors, including raises, bonuses, promotions, and in-house awards.

As James's narrative unfolded, it became clear that he was living out a story in which he lived alone, unconnected to and unsupported by any other human being. This state of affairs was explained on at least two levels of conscious articulation. Running through his story were emphatically felt, but only dimly perceived, notions of himself as defective, unlovable, and unwanted. Correspondingly, the significant figures in he life were depicted as hateful, self-involved, and totally unavailable. At a more distinct level of awareness, these key themes were buffered and hidden by a number of supporting ideologies and plots that justified that existence by glorifying it. That is, he chose to convince himself that his isolation, obsessive concern with work, and almost total lack of pleasure in life were desirable and superior ways of being. In particular, he construed these experiences as signs that he was coming close to achieving a mechanical, lifeless state that he had long glorified.

As James saw life, his only safety and protection came from the continual appeasement of his employers through his pursuit of professional perfection. His goal was to become a flawless "writing machine" that could work endlessly, effortlessly, and without any emotional or interpersonal encumbrances. In turn, because of his willingness to do more and more without complaint or protest, increasingly higher demands and expectations were placed on him. As a result, his search for perfection took on ironic coloration: The better he did at work, the more he doubted his ability to do well.

James portrayed himself as living without any deep emotional ties to other people, including his wife, two children, siblings, and parents. His description of his youth was the story of an isolated, unhappy, and eventually rebellious child and adolescent who learned to cope with his parents' anger, depression, and almost total unavailability by walling himself off in a world of literature, music, poetry, and hallucinogenic drugs. The unstated but intense purpose behind this immersion in imagination and the intellect was to aid in his quest for perfection, which he was later to learn was defined as total freedom from needing others and from being vulnerable in interpersonal relationships. As an adult, he had structured his life around this theme, most specifically in his choice of career. He found the subject matter appealing because it was factual, mechanical, and impersonal. However, beneath the surface of this story lay the seeds of his distress, in that he continued to need approval from parental surrogates (his employers), whom he perceived to be as implacable and unattainable as his parents.

Similarly, his lack of investment in his family life earned him the anger, disgust, and growing rejection of his wife and children. James had married a woman whom he consciously identified as being as entirely different from either of his parents as was possible: She was warm, comfortable with herself and with others, sexually passionate, and initially quite giving and supportive. However, in another ironic theme of his story, James had transformed his wife into a replica of his mother through his obsessive preoccupation with work. Her growing resentment, coldness, and distance, which were fueled by his physical and emotional absences, confirmed his portrayals of people as hurtful, unreliable, and abandoning. As importantly, the flaws in the marriage served to reinforce his sense of himself as unlovable and as existing in an emotional and interpersonal desert. The image of the "machine" to which he aspired had its underside: a set of interwoven images, beliefs, themes, and scripts in which he was cast as undesirable, defective, unlovable, and hopeless.

Running through James's story were a number of barely articulated but powerful, intense emotional states. These experiences were part of an alternative narrative that contained the makings of the life that James had hoped for but despaired of ever attaining. In this story, of which James had little awareness at the beginning of therapy, he was engaged in meaningful, creative, and self-expressive work as a writer of literature or poetry. This narrative also included the vision of satisfying relations with others, embedded in which were a sense of himself as a generous, concerned, joyous, and lovable, desirable person.

The despair that he felt about attaining this life was palpable to those around him, though he did not include that emotion in his consciousness. Instead, he dealt with it through a cynical, wisecracking, and somewhat contemptuous outlook on life (and psychotherapy). He discussed his parents in this framework and gradually revealed his defensive, compensatory construction of his history and development. In this story, his parents had played, and continued to play, little role in his emotional life. He envisioned himself as having transcended the need for parenting and for intimacy very early in life and was critical of and angry at others who had not reached such a state. In his view, his parents had done their best, and if that had not been very much, then so be it. After all, he had not been starved, beaten, sexually abused, or deprived of any physical comforts or social and educational opportunities. He argued strongly that he had taken nothing emotionally or psychological from his relationship with his parents; yet his descriptions of his interactions suggested an important identification with their frailties, fears, and behavior.

The anger, sadness, and hurt that were unvoiced parts of his descriptions of his earlier years had been unwittingly incorporated into his self-image. As he told it, he felt that meaningful relationships and work were impossible for him because "In those areas, everything I touch turns to garbage." His emotional life in general was flat and empty, save for brief moments of joy when he saw himself as becoming "more machinelike," and a pervasive fear and anxiety accompanied his search for perfection.

In spite of his extraordinary intellectual gifts and capacity, James suffered a number of cognitive and behavioral deficits. His ability to converse with other people in a comfortable and socially appropriate ways was very limited, as was his ability to evaluate his work, to soothe himself when he was strained or frightened, and to care for himself when he was tired or ill. His thinking and behavior were dominated by ideas and actions that served to heighten and accentuate his failures to reach perfection, while continuing to demand such attainments. These modes of functioning were incorporated into his narrative structure by way of reversal, in an attempt to turn difficulties into advantages. James managed his social anxieties and his disregard for his physical well-being by denigrating social life and the life of the body, and by describing to himself and to others the superiority of his intellectualized, work-obsessed approach to existence. Ironically, these attitudes duplicated his parents' social isolation and haughty disregard of others and, at the same time, were an enactment of their neglect of him as a child.

James's narrative was dominated by the ironic and tragic visions, which obscured and contained within them a latent romantic narrative. It was ironic because, in attempting to live life in a protected, mechanical way, he had demonstrated his parents' influence on him despite all his intentions to deny and escape that influence. The more machinelike he became, the more anxious and doubtful he felt. His repetition of his relationship to his parents in his marriage, with his increasingly demanding employers, in his unwitting living out of parental identifications, and in his hostile, neglectful approach to himself demonstrates both ironic and tragic elements. The irony lies in the repetition of a way of life that he despised and wished to escape; his search for perfection and for life as a machine never gained him the peace and security for which he sought. Instead, this search promoted and maintained the very anxiety and vulnerability it was meant to alleviate. The tragic pieces of James's story can be found in the determining power of pieces of the narrative of which he was almost totally unaware. There was a tremendous mismatch between the conscious aspects of James's story of his life and the actual ways in which he lived. This discrepancy, of course, reflected the living out of aspects of his history, early attachments, and enduring sense of pain, loss, and anger. Yet none of these factors were accorded much weight in the story of which he was aware. The latent romantic part was suggested by the palpable but unacknowledged longing for connection, meaning, and pleasure that could be inferred continually from James's participation in therapy. The romantic vision was also implied by the estrangement from self that much of his conscious narrative was intended to mask.

The comedic vision was neglected and actively denied in this story. In fact, it is possible to describe James's narrative as "countercomedic" in his insistence in isolating himself from the influences and impact of the external world and from emotional contact with others. Even so, the comedic vision was perceivable historically, with regard to the enduring impact of his early life, as well as the dimly realized aversion to interpersonal contact. This latter expressed in a disguised fashion James's sense of the possibility of external influences.

This summary cannot completely convey the complexity and nuances of James's narrative presentation. However, it does contain the main aspects of his construal of his life. The summary also points out how this ongoing story held within it the suffering that led him to seek therapy. In the chapters that follow, we will return to the narrative in more focused ways to illustrate its use as a foundation for an integrated psychotherapy.

3

Theories of
Psychotherapeutic Change

TRADITIONAL APPROACHES TO CHANGE

There are two broadly defined conceptualizations of change processes within current psychodynamic thinking. The first, which emphasizes insight into unconscious processes, is more traditional and is derived directly from Freud's earliest work in psychoanalysis (see Freud, 1894, 1898). The second view of change is considered to be more radical within the psychoanalytic world and is a result of the work of such revisionists as Alexander and French (1946), who stressed that new experience within therapy is central to changes in behavior, symptoms, character, and intrapsychic processes and structures.

Insight involves the patient's learning something specific about his or her unconscious psychological activity. The patient becomes aware of some forbidden, frightening, and painfully evocative wish, emotion, motive, fantasy, or memory that has been influencing his or her mental life in covert, powerful ways. Complete insight also contains the entrance into awareness of how the patient kept himself or herself unknowing (defense mechanisms, inhibitions, and character traits). The final component of insight involves learning about the anxieties, painful affects, self-images, and anticipated interpersonal consequences that led to the original warding off or disavowal of the particular issue. The emotional process of experiencing and integrating previously defended against conflicts is known as *abreaction* and

is always cited as critical to therapeutic change. Intellectual awareness of one's conflicts never leads to change without abreaction.

Insight and abreaction sometimes occur spontaneously as the patient associates freely in the presence of the therapist. Most often,
these experiences follow some interpretation offered by the psychoanalyst, in which the patient is told about the contents of the unconscious conflict, its historical roots, and its present-day
manifestations. An accurate interpretation seems to lead to the recovery of memories, to affective arousal, and to greater awareness of previously hidden feelings, desires, self-images, and object
representations. As these mental contents become conscious, the consequent anxiety, guilt, shame, or other affective correlates of those
inner states decrease. As insight and abreaction occur with some regularity over the course of therapy, the patient is freed of the burden-
some psychic task of drastically limiting his or her intrapsychic life
through defenses, symptoms, and distortions of behavior. Additionally, insight into problematic self-images and images of others that
are regressive and evocative of anxiety allows the person to revise
those representations and to form a more benign and productive representational system.

Insight is essentially an intrapsychic event that theoretically requires little interpersonal interchange (Greenberg & Mitchell, 1983).
However, since at least the 1930s, analysts have been aware that the
therapeutic interaction is at least as important as insight in promoting
change (see Strachey, 1934). This thesis was formulated most clearly
by Alexander and French (1946), who argued that a "corrective emotional experience" in psychoanalysis causes the patient to change. In
their view, insight follows intrapsychic and interpersonal change as
frequently as, or more frequently than, it precedes change.

The "corrective emotional experience" proposed by Alexander
and French (1946) is the forerunner of any number of psychoanalytic
concepts that describe the ways in which new, ameliorative experiences are provided for the patient by the therapist (for some examples
of these approaches, see the work of Kohut, 1977; Levenson, 1983;
Winnicott, 1971). Repetitive occurrences of empathy, soothing, encouragement, admiration, limit setting, or any other significant interpersonal events are translated into revised internal representations of
the self and of others. Essentially, the analyst interacts with the patient in ways that differ considerably from past interactions in which
the patient was slighted, hurt, abused, neglected, or made unable to
act as a unique individual. Such positive, novel experiences allow
gaps in the intrapsychic structure to be filled in through identification

with the positive attributes of the therapist. They also promote new and healthier ways of interacting with others. The therapist becomes the prototype for new representations of others that correct and replace fearsome, hateful, or ineffective object images, while the emotional sense of being responded to thoughtfully, sensitively, and compassionately becomes the core of a new, stable sense of the self and a new process of thinking about, and relating to, the self. Sometimes insight and historical reconstruction are antecedents to these interchanges, and often increased awareness by the patient of intrapsychic content occurs simultaneously with, or after, a corrective therapeutic exchange.

Humanistic, experiential, and existential psychotherapies share an emphasis on the importance of the provision of new experience by and with the therapist as the major component of change. New and ameliorative interactions are regarded as leading to an expansion and deepening of the patient's capacity to be aware of all aspects of experience, and to be more fully himself or herself in interpersonal situations that previously would have led to some distortion or shrinking of consciousness.

Rogers (1957) and other client centered therapists have identified three "necessary and sufficient" conditions for psychological growth in psychotherapy. These conditions are intrinsic facets of the therapeutic relationship: unconditional positive regard for the client, warmth, and accurate empathy. These relationship variables are communicated to the patient via reflection by the therapist of the client's latent or unsymbolized feelings. Thus, a fourth condition of change exists: the congruence of the therapist, which allows him or her to openly experience and accept the patient without any other agenda. In such an environment, the client's anxieties and uncertainties are markedly reduced. He or she is then gradually enabled to explore the moment-to-moment changes in affective, sensory, and cognitive experience that had previously been distorted or left unsymbolized. The safety and acceptance of the effective client-centered interaction allow the person to examine and to give up the socially conditioned facade that he or she has erected to feel secure. Full personhood (Rogers, 1961) is obtained slowly and is typified by the identification of an inner sense of directedness, wholeness, and an enhanced ability to symbolize and to integrate all aspects of experience.

The expansion of awareness, particularly of bodily and emotional needs and states, is the goal of Gestalt therapy and, as Perls (1973) demonstrated, is accomplished through a series of active exercises and confrontations. The mechanisms that are regarded as producing change involve the focusing of attention and awareness on the ways in which the person distorts, avoids, or transforms emotions, fantasies, desires, and bodily states. Attentional focusing, experiential exercises, and the resultant heightened awareness are presumed to eventuate in a conscious sense of the levels of faulty, self-estranged, and falsified modes of living that produce psychopathology. Authentic experience and an expansion of awareness emerge as the person becomes able to acknowledge his or her own role in limiting conscious experience, as well as the pain and anxiety that set such processes in motion, and is thus able gradually to accept spontaneous emotions, needs, and wishes.

Existential writers appear to be in great agreement with their client-centered and Gestalt colleagues in stressing the curative role of immediate, spontaneous, therapeutic experience (e.g., Bugenthal & Kleiner, 1993; Yalom, 1981). Existential therapy depends on active confrontation of the existential givens that the person fears and of the way in which she or he retreats into in authentic modes of experience in order to avoid responsibility. The interaction with the therapist is crucial in this regard. The therapist's confrontation of these in authentic patterns and processes, as well as his or her refusal to accept and participate in them, makes such activity more and more untenable. As a result, the person may come to an active decision to face his or her anxieties. Complete change occurs as these anxieties are faced, and accepted, with the result that important spheres of experience can be integrated. The relationship with the therapist is a critical factor in this process. Sharing one's distress with another who does not impose solutions or flee from the pain allows that other to be internalized as a schematic support with which the realities of life can be faced more openly. As the person admits both anxieties and potentials into her or his experience, a more genuine state of existence emerges, with a corresponding reduction in pathology.

Learning processes are the critical variable employed by cognitive-behavioral therapists, who emphasize the provision of novel experience as a necessary precondition for change. These therapies stress the correction of deviant behavioral and cognitive processes, as well as the gradual acquisition of productive, adaptive skills. Concepts drawn from social learning theory, cognitive psychology, and classical and operant conditioning form the theoretical framework for understanding how a person changes and improves through psychotherapy.

Many of the standard techniques of traditional behavior therapy, such as systematic desensitization, assertiveness training, or flooding, rely on processes of exposure and extinction to lessen anxious, phobic, or other fearful responses (Goldfried & Davison, 1976, 1994; Wolpe, 1958). Assisting a patient to gradually abandon a pattern of avoidance that is motivated by fear, and to face the internal or external stimuli that provoke that fear, is perhaps the most frequently relied-upon change principle in this group of interventions. Operant principles of positive and negative reinforcement, habituation, and shaping also play a frequent and important role in promoting exposure, and in building up new, adaptive patterns of thinking and of action. Social learning through the observation of effective models is an essential part of such techniques as behavior rehearsal, social skills training, communication training, and parent training, to name only a few. This type of learning effectively corrects deviant actions, allows the acquisition of new behaviors to replace or to fill in deficits, and is also an aid in promoting exposure and reduction of anxiety.

More cognitively oriented therapies rely heavily on the learning principles just described, but they add to this mix a powerful focus on the acquisition of new ways of perceiving and thinking about experience, as well as the correction and modification of dysfunctional beliefs, attitudes, and ideas. Most descriptions of cognitive therapy stress the role of experiential learning as a critical change factor: The patient experiences in an immediate way the impact of particular thoughts and perceptions and then learns from the therapist's ways to test, evaluate, and correct those cognitions. Modification of dysfunctional cognition therefore depends on a shift in set about one's psychological processes, and on the possession or development of the ability to reflect on, and to report about, inner states. This ability to think about psychological events has been called *psychological-mindedness or metacognition.*

Cognitive-behavioral therapies strongly place action, repetition, and practice at the center of therapeutic gain. Awareness without behavioral change (insight) is viewed as having little, if any, therapeutic impact. Insight is frequently described as a correlate or consequence of newly acquired or changed behavior, rather than as a cause of improvement.

New experience becomes the basic stuff of restructured patterns of interpersonal relatedness, and of revised and more open representational structures. Deep change is considered a desirable and significant goal in these therapies. It is an indirect goal that follows from, and is based on, the patient's enhanced ability to live capably and successful, following new learning and the reduction of psychopathology.

INTEGRATIVE THEORIES OF CHANGE

Two broad classes of models of change within psychotherapy integration may be identified. These two groupings correspond with the level of integration that is represented: the common-factors approach to integration and the theoretical integration of therapies.

Within the common-factors class, studies of change processes have attempted to identify those variables of psychological influence that are common to most or all therapies (Weinberger, 1993; see also Chapter 1). This work follows on the pioneering efforts of such writers as Rosenzweig (1936), Alexander and French (1946), Shoben (1949), Dollard and Miller (1950), and most important, Frank (1961). These efforts stress the role of the provision of new and benign interpersonal experience within an accepting relationship with a healer, one that is sanctioned and guided by a rationale for regular interaction and for efforts at change. Frank's (1961) cross-cultural common-factors studies of psychotherapy remain a landmark in this field. He identified the provision of hope, of an expectation of change, and of a sense of effectiveness and well-being as the central, common-factors of change in psychotherapy and in folk healing. The therapeutic relationship, with its socially condoned and empowered aura, its regularity of contact, and its techniques and rituals, may elicit these attitudinal changes in the patient. Such changes in the person's affective and cognitive state may be of enormous assistance in enabling that individual to make further behavioral and intrapsychic changes (Weinberger, 1993).

More contemporary integrative studies of therapeutic change have confirmed and expanded on these early findings. For example, Strupp (1971) suggested that improvement in psychotherapy is brought about by three central factors: The positive alliance that develops between patient and therapist provides hope and an expectation of change and serves as a power base for the next two factors. All therapies contain some methods of interpersonal influence that are based on covert or explicit ideologies, and that can work only because of the alliance between the two participants. The last factor cited by Strupp (1971) is the patient's willingness and capacity to put into everyday use the new learning and experience that have been provided by the therapeutic interaction.

Orlinsky and Howard (1986) wrote about a similar set of components of therapeutic influence: the therapeutic contract, interventions that are prescribed and sanctioned by that contract, the bond between patient and therapist, the degree to which the patient's experience of his or her participation in therapy is marked by openness or defensiveness (termed *patient self-relatedness*), and the realizations or gains generated by therapeutic contact.

Goldfried (1980, 1982, 1983, 1995) has argued cogently for locating common change factors at the level of clinical strategies and principles. He suggested that this approach will maximize the ability of therapists of different orientations to communicate about their therapies, and to compare these therapies effectively.

Goldfried (1982, 1983) identified the induction of positive, hopeful expectations for change as one common strategy that cuts across all psychotherapies. The other strategies are the provision of a secure and humane therapeutic relationship; the provision of feedback and an external perspective on the patient's problems by the therapist; a focus on corrective, novel experiences in and out of sessions; and repeated chances for revision of one's construction of reality.

Arkowitz and Hannah (1989) integrated Goldfried's work on clinical strategies with Alexander and French's (1946) concept of the corrective emotional experience to develop a common-factors theory of change that stresses the central role of *behavioral enactment*. They define this term as the demonstration of the patient's problem, in all of its intrapsychic, cognitive, behavioral, and affective components, in some interpersonal interaction. Such enactments can occur in or out of therapy. In the context of appropriate emotional arousal, new responses to the enactment by the therapist and by significant others in the patient's life may lead to disconfirmation of the representational underpinnings of that problem. Such work is viewed as cutting across all therapeutic boundaries.

Recent and comprehensive reviews of the common-factors literature by Grencavage and Norcross (1990) and Weinberger (1993, 1995) seem to capture the current state of integrative change models. Grencavage and Norcross (1990) found that six change factors are typically cited in the clinical literature: a therapeutic alliance marked by trust, openness, warmth, and gradually increasing levels of self-revelation by the patient; periodic expressions of painful and previously avoided emotions (catharsis); the shaping and practice of new skills and behaviors, particularly in areas of fear or of interpersonal deficits; the provision of hope and of positive expectations for change; the ameliorative and beneficial characteristics of the therapist, especially with regard to his or her ability to encourage the patient to be optimistic and hopeful; and the presence of a therapeutic ideology or rationale that explains the patient's suffering and prescribes methods for improvement.

Weinberger (1993, 1995) examined the empirical status of this list of change factors and concluded that there is modest but incomplete, somewhat vague research support for these factors in general, but that some of these change components do stand up to empirical test. In particular, Weinberger (1993) noted that corrective experiences that expose the patient to a previously avoided fear and/or are emotionally charged and cathartic have been documented repeatedly to be beneficial to the patient. Similarly, he cited the work of Bandura (1977, 1982) on self-perception and self-efficacy as demonstrating the power of changing the patient's expectations. As Weinberger (1993) noted, Bandura (1982) argued that enhanced self-efficacy is the single most powerful change factor in all therapies and seems to define operationally the notions of remoralization and hope identified by Frank (1961) and his successors.

A number of modern integrative psychotherapies are built around common-factors theories of psychological change. They all start from the premise that the generic, relationship-derived factors identified by Frank (1961, see above) are powerfully operative. However, the creators of these systems do not wish to rely on these change processes, which are fairly vague and are difficult to operationalize and to activate systematically. Instead, these common-factors theories of change, and the associated therapies, represent efforts to combine and to maximize the range of effective therapeutic interventions and experiences that are available to any patient. Typically, each system provides an assessment framework into which the patient's symptoms, personality traits, environment, and history may be fitted. Out of this assessment comes a recommended sequence of interventions that reflects the unique combination of change factors that appear to be best suited to the patient's needs.

Among the common-factors theories of change in this branch of psychotherapy integration, Prochaska's transtheoretical model (1995; Prochaska & DiClemente, 1992a, b) is the most often cited and the most comprehensive description of the multitude of active change processes in psychotherapy. His common-factors analysis of a variety of psychotherapeutic systems led him to identify 10 common change processes, and to formulate a five-stage theory of psychotherapeutic change. Each stage is marked by the patient's relationship to and perception of his or her problems. A relationship exists between the stage of change and the necessary psychological processes that may produce change. Movement within each stage and between stages is determined by one or several of the 10 change factors. The change factors identified are:

1. Consciousness raising
2. Self-liberation
3. Social liberation
4. Counterconditioning
5. Stimulus control
6. Self-reevalution
7. Environmental reevaluation
8. Contingency management
9. Dramatic relief
10. Helping relationships (from Prochaska & DiClemente, 1992b, p. 302)

The earliest stage of change is *precontemplation.* In this stage, the person is unconscious of or unable or unwilling to discuss a particular problem. Change is construed as having more negative consequences than would the continuation of the problem. Consciousness raising and reevaluation of the self and the environment are the necessary experiences for movement to the next stage. The therapeutic techniques of the dynamic, humanistic, and cognitive therapies are useful at this point.

Contemplation involves a cognitive and affective review of a problem, a search for new data, and an open consideration of the consequences of change. Progress at this stage depends on self-evaluation, environmental evaluation, emotional relief, and helping relationships. Once again, cognitive, analytic, and experiential work can activate these processes.

Preparation is the next stage of change, and progress here is based on the processes of continued self-evaluation and of self-liberation. The person engages in activities that indicate a readiness for action and for overt behavioral change. Preparation for change seems to be an active ingredient of Gestalt work, cognitive restructuring, existential therapy, and systems models.

The amelioration of symptoms and the modification of problematic behaviors occur in the stage of *action.* In this stage, traditional behavioral and cognitive change processes and techniques most obviously employed are contingency management, stimulus control, and counterconditioning.

The final stage of change is the *maintenance* stage. Gains are consolidated, and complex interpersonal and intrapersonal relationships are restructured to allow new and positively reinforcing cycles to develop. Any therapeutic intervention may be part of the work at this level.

A third part of this theory of change is the assessment of the psychological level or sphere of problematic functioning (Prochaska & DiClemente, 1992b). These levels include symptoms or situational difficulties, maladaptive cognitions, interpersonal conflicts, family systems conflicts, and intrapsychic conflicts. Problems that occur in these different areas of life may require interventions drawn from one or two of the several therapies that are broadly appropriate to the stage of change, and to the necessary mechanisms of change. For example, work on dysfunctional patterns of thinking at the precontemplation level of change may respond best to techniques from Adlerian therapy, while modification of such problems would proceed most effectively with cognitive therapy techniques if the patient were at the stage of preparation or action. The underlying change mechanisms in both cases would be consciousness raising, self-reevaluation, and environmental reevaluation.

Other important, integrative common-factors theories of change resemble the transtheoretical model but select somewhat different processes for emphasis. Garfield (1992) suggested that the corrective impact of a safe, warm, and accepting therapeutic relationship is a precondition for all other therapeutic change. He cited emotional release, insight, provision of explanations for disturbed behavior, desensitization through exposure, operant conditioning, and skills training as the major change processes in therapy. Beitman (1992) saw exposure to feared, painful, and avoided psychological states and interpersonal situations as the central change factors that cut across most psychotherapies. He radically redefined exposure broadly and inclusively, suggesting that it occurs both through techniques that explicitly aim at exposure, and through a variety of other experiences. In the first group are such behavioral interventions as systematic and *in vivo* desensitization, flooding assertiveness training, and response prevention. However, Beitman pointed out that such interventions as directive instruction, insight, grief work, social skills training, and modification of interpersonal patterns all require and cause the person to expose himself or herself to inner and outer events that have been uncomfortable, difficult, or frightening.

Beutler (Beutler & Consoli, 1992; Beutler & Hodgson, 1993) based his prescriptive, technically eclectic approach to psychotherapy integration on an explicit amalgam of Beitman's (1992) and Prochaska and DiClemente's (1992a, b) models of change. His unique contribution is the careful, empirically based matching procedure employed when one is selecting techniques. Beutler's work offers the therapist a detailed and practical guide to maximizing change at any level and stage of the patient's functioning.

In the most general terms, theoretical integration stresses the contribution and mutual interplay of expanded awareness and the corrective experience in and out of therapy, within the setting of a positively toned, safe, and accepting therapeutic relationship. Expanded awareness sometimes leads to change; at other times, it serves as a map or signpost to alert the patient to the need for overt actions and new learning (Fisch, Weakland, & Segal, 1982; Westerman, 1993). In the view of writers who have argued for the theoretical integration of psychotherapies, improvement in psychological functioning is the result of increased freedom from self-defeating, ironic, and self-reinforcing intrapsychic and interpersonal patterns (see Fensterheim, 1993; Gold & Wachtel, 1993; Ryle, 1990; Safran & Segal, 1990; Westerman, 1993). These psychotherapies are attempts to add technical specificity and potency to the generic common change-factors and relationship variables that were described above. These writers have focused on the core group of processes that are most effective in highlighting and modifying the patient's disturbed relationships with himself or herself and with others. The interpersonally derived, nonspecific relationship factors (such as remoralization and the provision of hope) identified by others are endorsed by theoretical integrationists as well but are generally assumed to be a backdrop and foundation for work with specific change factors. These include exposure to anxiety-generating internal states and external situations, insight, modification of excessive or deviant responding through operant and classical conditioning principles, shaping of adaptive behavior patterns, and heightened emotional experience. These mechanisms can be ends in themselves, as in the traditional therapies from which they are drawn. More important, in these integrative models, any change process can be understood as a potential source of interruption or correction of an ironic, maladaptive circle.

The various models of theoretically integrated therapy rely on one or several of these change principles more heavily than on others. The reason is the specific construction of the maladaptive circles, and of the experiences that are necessary to correct those circles. For example, the active self model (Andrews, 1993) and cyclical psychodynamic therapy (Gold & Wachtel, 1993; Wachtel, 1993) give equal weight to the psychodynamic, behavioral, interpersonal, and affective components of pathological circles. Therefore, insight, deconditioning through exposure, social learning, and heightened emotionality are seen as equivalent in terms of general therapeutic potency. These processes are employed on a case-by-case basis, as the clinical needs of the individual dictate. Other systems of theoretical integration emphasize exposure above all other factors in leading to change. Examples include implosive therapy (Stampfl & Levis, 1967) and behavioral psychotherapy (Fensterheim, 1993). These therapies are built around the notion that exposure to, and deconditioning of, the anxiety associated with underlying psychodynamic conflicts is the most important source of therapeutic change. Other change factors are relied on as necessary to promote the patient's willingness and ability to face previously avoided fears. Still other integrative models emphasize the combination of cognitive restructuring with corrective emotional and interpersonal interactions as the source of the most important therapeutic gains (Ryle, 1990; Safran & Segal, 1990). This emphasis follows from the theoretical weight given to disturbed cognition and its interpersonal manifestations and reinforcements. In these therapies, insight and other change processes are seen as useful, but as subsidiary.

A central point to be gleaned from this discussion is that circular theories of integration tend to include change processes in similar, circular, and novel ways. For example, in most of these therapies, insight and exposure are described as two sides of the same coin and, often, as possible only in the context of a new and corrective relationship (for theoretical and clinical illustrations of these points, see Fensterheim 1993; Gold & Wachtel, 1993). All of these therapies ultimately share a constructivistic or hermeneutic position on change, be it implied or overt, in that they aim to help the patient to rid himself or herself of old and pathogenic meanings, representations, and constructions of experience. As such meanings are jettisoned, opportunities for new representations of the self, others, and the environment may be provided and used. In this framework, all of the change processes discussed by the common-factors group and the theoretical integration contingent can be seen as subordinate or as parts of a larger and varied whole.

The most explicit focus on the reorganization of the patient's representational system as the central ameliorative process in psychotherapy is contained in the work of Greenberg (Greenberg et al., 1993; Watson & Greenberg, 1994), Guidano (1987, 1991; Guidano & Liotti, 1983), Horowitz (1988), Safran (Safran & Segal, 1990), Mahoney (1991), and Shapiro (Shapiro, Barkham, Reynolds, Hardy, & Stiles, 1992).

These authors have placed other change processes, including insight, cognitive restructuring, social learning, exposure, and a supportive therapeutic relationship, in an intermediate position with regard to the goal of deep structural change in the meanings that organize the person's experience and behavior. Any therapeutic activity is aimed simultaneously at two ends: change in the immediate psychological status of the patient and, more important, the provision of new experience that can be assimilated into the cognitive and affective matrix of schemas or of self- and object representations. Mahoney (1991) identified a number of change processes that are implicated in giving up old meanings and constructions and in generating a more useful ontological structure. Each of these processes can be derived from a variety of traditional and integrative therapeutic interventions. Essentially, he suggested that all effective therapeutic techniques lead to change by gradually challenging the person's existing modes of organizing experience. This confrontation promotes a state of disequilibrium that opens the person to new experience and to revision of the self-concept, images of others, and plans and strategies for adaptation. Guidano's (1987) description of his integrative therapy echoes Mahoney's vision of the deep changes in meanings that arise as the therapist challenges the patient's existing point of view.

Shapiro (Shapiro, Barkham, Reynolds, Hardy, & Stiles, 1992) utilized a Piagetian cognitive-developmental theory of the stages and processes of change to integrate prescriptive (cognitive-behavioral) and exploratory (psychodynamic) therapies. The ultimate goal of this treatment is the assimilation of problematic, unintegrated experience into the patient's existing schematic structures. As existing meanings and cognitive structures are expanded and modified by this process, pathogenic schemas can be corrected and replaced by adaptive meanings. Psychodynamic insight is most effective when the patient is unaware of the experiences and meanings that need to be assimilated. Problems that are already known to the patient can be addressed through anxiety management techniques, cognitive restructuring, self-management work, and stress reduction techniques. Greenberg and his colleagues (Greenberg et al., 1993; Watson & Greenberg, 1994) have also aimed at schematic restructuring as the final and most important goal of their integrative, experientially based psychotherapy. They have identified seven phases of the change process, each of which requires a different level and type of intervention. The first phase, building a relationship, is the foundation of all later work and also serves to alleviate a good deal of the patient's distress by pro-

viding support and acceptance. In the next phase, empathic exploration, problematic aspects of the patient's experience are identified and
are targeted for intervention in the subsequent phases. The next three
stages (task initiation, evocation and arousal, and experiential exploration) involve active work within problem areas through the use of
techniques derived from experiential and Gestalt therapies. This work
leads to a better differentiation of the patient's experience and emotional life, the giving up of unfinished business with others from the
past, and the next phases of change. This phase involves schematic
change. It results from the interplay of the emotional, cognitive, and
behavioral changes, which accrued in the earlier phases, with an expanded ability and investment in self-examination, and in reconstrual
of interpersonal relations and the environment. Such modifications
in deep structures of organizing experience then result in new, creative, and adaptive life plans and decisions.

The ironic, self-confirming, and self-protective role of representational structures has been recognized by all of the authors cited
above. Deep structural changes in how any person finds and organizes
meanings do not come without much conflict and pain. Often, it is
impossible to separate deeply held meanings from the person's central
sense of selfhood and identity (Guidano, 1987; Mahoney, 1991). As
a result, examination of the ways in which a person struggles to protect, preserve, and maintain her or his modes of construing experience is crucial in integrative approaches to the phenomena of
resistance, reactance, transference, and countertransference. It is inevitable that the therapist will become embroiled in the patient's enactments, symptoms, and ironic patterns of pathology. Interactions
become the source of many opportunities for the kinds of change
experiences that have been described in this chapter. However, such
patterns of relating also make up the chief source of therapeutic
blockages and stalemates (see Chapter 4).

A NARRATIVE-BASED SYNTHESIS OF
INTEGRATIVE THEORIES OF CHANGE

The discussion just concluded seems to suggest that, if all roads
don't lead to Rome, a great many of them do. Psychological change
is the end product of travel down a large number of parallel pathways. On each path, the significant experiences one encounters may
be different to a greater or lessor degree. Yet these adventures appear

to conclude, when successful, with the person's life having been altered in many of the same ways as are the lives of his or her fellow travelers who took other trails.

The narrative model of personality and psychopathology that was proposed in the last chapter allows us to unify the integrative work on psychological change. Each patient comes to therapy because of suffering that can ultimately be traced to a faulty, "broken," or inappropriate narrative. These precursors of psychopathology will of course be faulty in overlapping but somewhat different ways for each person. Similarly, the narrative foundation will contain differing positive aspects across different patients, resulting in the variety of unique adaptive skills, strengths, and potentials that make up each person's individuality. Finally, every patient has a personal, unique, and critically important relationship to his or her narrative constructions of experience. Some people are totally unaware of the story that they have developed and are living out, while others are full cognizant of their worldview, scripts, and plots. Most people fall somewhere between these two extremes.

Additionally the relationship to one's narrative contains some conscious and unwitting attitudes and beliefs about the role and influence of that complex story line in determining the person's behavior, experience, and distress. Again, individual perceptions of this process vary greatly, from those who see no connection between their psychological life and its narrative framework to some who are fully immersed in that story and its ramifications and consequences. We can find in this description similarities to the stages of change work of Prochaska (Prochaska & DiClemente, 1992a, b) and the other authors cited above. Prochaska's initial changes (precontemplation and contemplation) indicate a relatively unformulated relationship with one's own story, possibly one in which that narrative is accorded little weight in determining the person's life path. A well-developed internal sense of the place of one's narrative in behavior and experience would seem to place the person at the later stages of change.

The path to change is also determined by the specific parts of the narrative that are working, and by those that are not. Unformulated narratives or pieces of narrative correspond to the unconscious or unsymbolized aspects of psychological life that are the focus of psychodynamic, humanistic, and experiential therapies. When a patient is "being lived by" his or her story without knowing it, insight and the expansion of awareness are critical components of any desired change. This alteration of the patient's approach to the narrative must also include an increased awareness of the reasons, past and present, interpersonal and intrapersonal, why some aspects of the narrative were kept out of the story.

Faulty subplots, scripts, or characterizations of the self and other do not often change through insight alone. Narratives are held onto stubbornly and adamantly. As such integrative writers as Guidano (1987, 1991) and Mahoney (1991) have pointed out, change in basic representational models may be resisted because of the potential loss of identity and security that such change often suggests. Often, new and corrective experience must precede any loosening of the central pathogenic narrative units. The patient must experience fully, with heightened affect and full awareness, the impact of the existing stories about the self and others. He or she may be able to change those stories if new experiences demonstrate, immediately and powerfully, the utility of revisions. The new experiences that will be helpful to any particular person will depend on the parts of the story that cause the person to get into trouble. Faulty aspects of a narrative may reveal themselves through difficulties with the integration or modulation of emotions, through cognitive distortions or deficits, or through behavioral excesses, gaps, or deviations. Directive work with these disturbances through cognitive, behavioral, or experiential techniques not only will enhance the patient's functioning but will increase his or her ability to contact new experiences and thus to confront, examine, and modify the existing narrative. Each behavioral, cognitive, or affective change that accrues may be integrated into the person's story about the self (self-image or representation). As that story line is altered, the person may become more ready and able to approach other people differently. As new experiences accumulate, modifications in interpersonal scripts and plots may be seen as possible and desirable. As a result, the tragic and ironic consequences of the original narrative will decrease or end (see Chapter 2).

Significant people in the patient's life often have overt, unconscious, or unintended investments in her or his dysfunctional tale. For example, the spouse of a man who tells the story of himself as stupid and unable to think clearly may use that narrative to heighten her sense of intelligence and superiority. Such an accomplice (Gold & Wachtel, 1993; Wachtel, 1993) can wreck the efforts of even the best therapy. If this is the case, work on limiting the impact of the accomplice by systemic, behavioral, or interpersonal training may be of foremost importance.

The therapeutic relationship is crucial to any narrative reconstruction. The narratives initially brought to therapy by patients are often devoid of hope or of a portrayal of themselves as competent and effective. The decision to begin treatment may be the last gasp of optimism, or the first sign of the stirrings of hope. The acceptance, warmth, prizing, and empathy offered by the therapist can have a major impact on the patient's story in a number of ways. First, such positive responses will evoke those aspects of the patient's self-image that are in need of revision and may provide some of the raw material for such alteration. The ways in which the patient is unable or unwilling, because of historical issues or current conflicts, to use a positive reception by the therapist for such revisions also become apparent. The therapist's actions, attitudes, and ways of relating will highlight critical interpersonal stories and scripts. Again, this material may allow the patient to change certain ideas about other people or may point out in a highly charged way the ironic patterns of interpersonal interaction that reinforce and maintain certain crucial story lines. Finally, the task of exposing oneself to warded-off components of a narrative and to the new experiences that are necessary to change that narrative requires great courage and dedication (Fried, 1983). The support, encouragement, guidance, and companionship of the therapist help ease the fear of the patient and may bolster his or her sense of self-efficacy and boldness in facing the unknown.

CASE EXAMPLE: JAMES

The ways in which James's pathogenic narrative became the focus of an integrative psychotherapy are explored in much detail in Chapters 4, 5, 6, and 7. In these discussions, the impact on his ongoing story of the therapeutic relationship, of insight, of action-oriented interventions, and of the generation of emotional experience is explored. In concluding this chapter, we briefly return to the central themes in James's tale and identify the critical change processes and events that those elements seemed to require.

James's initial approach to therapy was organized around his portrayal of himself as a machine, one that needed no one, could be influenced by no other person, and one whose goals were antithetical to the therapeutic process. He was skeptical about the theories and methods of psychotherapy and often spent much time and effort reporting on his views about the neurochemical etiology of his problems. James's representation of himself as standing outside the realm of interpersonal need, contact, or assistance was therefore the first element of the story that needed to be addressed. This view of his

existence and experience served as a major resistance against allowing the therapy and the therapist to become meaningful aspects of
his psychological life and helped James to repress or disown the
other, more deeply disturbing, subplot in his tale: that of someone
whose hopes for contact and intimacy were doomed to fail because
of his destructive effects on relationships.

Thus, James began therapy at a point of potential change that
fell within the precontemplative phase (Prochaska & DiClemente,
1992a). It seemed necessary and appropriate, therefore, to work psychodynamically in order to understand the meaning of this story to
James, it protective role in his emotional life, and his attachments to
this part of the narrative. Additionally, an empathic, warm, interested,
and prizing stance was taken with him, even as he battled with the
therapist by criticizing, debating, and retreating into his intellect.
These interventions and their effects on James and his narrative structure are discussed at much greater length in later chapters. Here, it
suffices to suggest that the combination of empathic understanding
and insight into the unconscious meaning and role of his "machine
story" led James to make an important attachment to the therapy and
the work of the treatment. As he became aware of these investments,
the subtext of "Everything I touch turns to garbage" emerged into
James's awareness. This theme and James's gradual and highly pained
owning of it seemed to indicate that he had moved into the change
stages of contemplation and action, and it led to work (also described
in later chapters) with a variety of behavioral, cognitive, and experiential interventions. Additionally, the therapeutic relationship continued to provide new material about his worth as a person, his need
of and desire for contact and closeness, and his transferential ways
of avoiding or denying those needs.

Change is never straightforward, and it certainly was not easy
for James. He moved from one aspect of the narrative to the other,
and his ability to connect to the important themes and to the required
work varied greatly, as it does in all therapies. Over time, as he became more confident in himself and in his capacity to love and to
be loved, the therapy moved onto a dual thematic track. The older
themes of "machine" and "interpersonal garbage maker" continued
to sound, but in more muted and less influential ways. New stories
and scripts emerged that contained fragile, hopeful, and positive
views of his chances in life; his capabilities as father, husband, and
friend; his role in his company and in the world of poetry and literature; and his connection to the therapist. Also, he began to rewrite
his history and the story of his family life in more complete, emo-

tionally poignant, and complex ways that admitted his lost chances for closeness, the sadness and anger that had accompanied those experience, and the ways in which his parents had both done well by him and had failed him.

In order to be facilitated, completed, and reinforced, these narrative shifts required work at all levels of psychological life: affective, cognitive, behavioral, and psychodynamic. Much time and effort were spent examining the therapeutic relationship with regard to its role as a source of new portrayals of the self and of others. James's new story was more open, tentative, benign, and creative than the narrative with which he had started therapy. It enabled him to realize some of his hopes for satisfaction and security personally and professionally but also forced him to be receptive to life's pain and disappointments, from which he had successfully protected himself in the past through his "machine" story. It was this type of change that most of the final interventions were aimed at.

II

Clinical Concepts

The Therapeutic Relationship

It is the rare student of therapy who would disagree with the notion that the interactive or interpersonal aspect of psychotherapy is critical at the levels of theory, observation, clinical understanding, and intervention. Yet, just as we currently lack a unified model of pathology or intervention, we miss a common and open construal of the meaning, process, and utility of the therapeutic relationship.

In some psychotherapies, integrative or otherwise, the conception of the relationship defines and structures how way technique, process, and change are considered, sought after, and evaluated. Other schools of psychotherapy suggest that the therapeutic interaction is more of a dependent variable, and that its evolution and course are determined by interventive and technical issues. Finally, certain therapists (especially those in the humanistic-experiential camp and others who adhere to the model proposed by Frank, 1961) argue that therapy is a relationship and that the two concepts cannot be separated in any significant way. The discussion that follows will examine this debate as well, in terms of the positions taken by writers within the integrative movement, and for its implications for future models of unified psychotherapy.

TRADITIONAL DEFINITIONS OF THE ROLES OF PATIENT AND THERAPIST

Almost all traditional psychotherapies cast the patient in the role of a seeker of help. This role definition is inevitable and probably is necessary for therapy to exist at all. Once the starting point of treatment has passed, with the establishment of a therapeutic agreement or contract, each therapy assigns its own unique tasks, goals, and responsibilities to the patient. However, patients in psychodynamic psychotherapy, humanistic therapy, and cognitive-behavioral therapy do share a common role definition beyond that of help seeker: They are defined as participants in a learning process. The unique styles and educational contents that define each sectarian school of psychotherapy, in turn, further define and refine the patient's specific role in those therapies.

Therapeutic stance (Gold, 1990b, 1993c) refers to the interpersonal positions, responsibilities, and activities that define and frame the interaction between patient and therapist. Ideas about the desired stance have prescriptive and preemptive aspects, in that each therapy describes the optimal role for the two participants by demanding certain behaviors and by forbidding others. Stance does not refer specifically to the content of therapy or to technical issues. Instead, it is the foundation on which all other therapeutic activities are based. Certain techniques and concepts are linked intrinsically to particular types of role definitions in psychotherapy and are contraindicated by other preferred stances. For example, the instructional efforts of cognitive-behavioral therapists are consistent with the teacher–student stance that is preferred by many therapists in that group. Yet such work cannot easily be accommodated by the stances that are preferred by humanistic and dynamic therapists. These stances are based openly on the avoidance of any attempts by the therapist to influence the patient directly or to change his or her behavior. The irreconcilable differences between the stances of the major schools of traditional psychotherapy are cited frequently by critics of psychotherapy integration. These differences are taken as proof of the impossibility of bridging the technical and conceptual gaps between the different systems.

Patients in psychoanalytically oriented therapies are engaged in the process of learning about their developmental histories; their unconscious motivations, conflicts, and defenses; and the ways in which they unwittingly intermingle and confuse the past and the present. It is the patient's explicit task to free-associate, that is, to act as an unfettered and open observer and reporter of his or her thoughts, feelings, images, sensations, and memories. These intrapsychic data are offered to the analyst as raw material for interpretations of the underlying meanings, fears, and wishes. It is assumed that the patients will eventually, learn to understand their own symbols and unconscious mental life on their own. Patient and therapist are seen as sharing the understanding that this process will lead, eventually and indirectly, to the alleviation of the suffering that brought the patient to therapy in the first place.

In more classically oriented analytic therapies, the therapist is advised to follow Freud's (1912) metaphor of surgical anonymity in conducting therapy. This metaphor suggests that a task focus is essential to the process, and that the therapist's personal issues, private life, and human desires are best left out of the consulting room. As Freud (1913) famously put it, the analyst must be "free of the desire to cure." This metaphor defines the individuality of the therapist as potentially disruptive to the process of understanding the deeper contents and structure of the patient's mind. Should the analyst move out of the role of the anonymous, interpreting observer, this position argues, his or her participation would contaminate the patient's associations. This Freudian model is based on the assumption that the mind is a closed system and that reality factors in and outside therapy are largely unimportant in personality development, in the etiology of psychopathology, and in the cure of neurosis.

As newer and more interpersonally oriented versions of psychoanalysis have emerged, so have newer, participatory definitions of the roles of patient and therapist. While the patient is involved in the analytic process to learn about his or her unconscious mental life, he or she is also often meant to have novel and corrective experiences with the analyst. In turn, the analyst is defined as a "participant observer" (Sullivan, 1953), and as the potential provider of a host of experiences that will counteract early parental failures and trauma (Mitchell, 1993). In this frame of reference, it is the therapists' task to understand and interpret the patient's verbal associations while monitoring and adjusting his or her own overall interaction with the patient. As Wolstein (1990) described this change in the analytic relationship, the therapist becomes an "observing participant" whose individuality and interpersonal skills are central to the process. Anonymity and an absence of personal involvement are deemed to be both impossible and therapeutically undesirable, in that the ongoing interaction between patient and therapist contains the raw material for new identifications, internalizations, and the building of healthy intrapsychic structures (Kohut, 1980; Mitchell, 1994).

In humanistic and experiential therapies, the patient is also seen as being involved in an intrapsychically oriented learning process. However, in these therapies, he or she receives an education about how his or her experience is distorted and constricted, and about the specific types of experiential events that are avoided or are left un-symbolized. The patient is regarded as being in charge of the explo-ration process, with the therapist serving as facilitator or consultant (Bugenthal & Kleiner, 1993; Rogers, 1959). It is the patient's job to dwell in the moment-to-moment stream of conscious experience and to describe as freely as possible the shifts, openings, and blockages in his or her awareness of bodily, psychological, and interpersonal experience. Therapists of these schools are advised to avoid the pre-sumption that they can ever know as much as or more than the pa-tient when it comes to the patient's experiences. This perspective rules out interpretive work and places the therapist in the role of coparticipant: The therapist reports his or her experiences with and of the patient to the patient or, particularly in Gestalt therapy, sug-gests exercises that may help the patient to undo a blockage.

Client-centered therapists have long been clear about their view that therapy and the therapeutic relationship are one and the same thing (Rogers, 1961). That is, the patient is healed by the encounter with a congruent, unconditionally prizing, and empathic individual. As this interaction proceeds, the patient is able to free himself or herself of the internal knots in which he or she was tied in adapting to a compromised environment. Neither Gestalt nor existential thera-pies equate therapy with the relationship as does client-centered ther-apy. However, virtually all humanistic and experiential therapies suggest that the psychological health and availability of the therapist are an indispensable component of therapeutic gain (Rice & Green-berg, 1992). Thus, a central part of the therapist's role is to remain self-involved while simultaneously communing with the patient. This self-focus resembles a tightrope act in its delicate balance. The thera-pist must monitor his or her own experience both to remain a source of data about the patient's unacknowledged feelings and thoughts and also avoid or correct reactions that are inauthentic or unempathic. Disregard of the therapist's ongoing reactions will impair progress, as will too much introspection.

Cognitive-behavioral therapies explicitly equate the therapist with the expert teacher and the patient with the student role. As Goldfried and Davison (1976) and Beck, Rush, Shaw, and Emory (1979), among many others, have pointed out, the cognitive-behav-ioral approach is instructional and didactic and relies heavily on the patient's active involvement in the learning process.

Most contemporary therapists of this school strongly emphasize the collaborative, Socratic nature of the teaching and learning process (see Beck, Freeman, et al., 1989). In this model, the therapist teaches the patient to experiment, to question, to act, and to evaluate, rather than rigidly offering prepackaged answers and solutions. The establishment of true collaboration depends on the therapist's being able to respect the patient and his or her strengths and abilities. A collaborative cognitive-behavioral therapist must not be invested in being the authority and must be quite willing to attribute a significant amount of expertise to the patient. At times, this means conceding that the patient knows more about his or her life, problems, assets, and disadvantages than does the therapist, or that the therapist's suggestions, teachings, and perspectives may be incorrect or useless.

Casting the patient in the role of collaborator also places heavy demands for activity and effort on his or her shoulders. The patient's willingness to try out techniques, particularly in out-of-session homework assignments, is crucial to the success of cognitive-behavioral work. Passivity and inactivity on the patient's part are countertherapeutic and may be a major source of resistance (see below).

TRADITIONAL CONCEPTUALIZATIONS OF THE THERAPEUTIC RELATIONSHIP

Psychoanalytic therapies divide the interaction between patient and therapist into three overlapping components: the "real relationship," the therapeutic alliance, and the transference–countertransference relationship. The "real" relationship consists of the social aspects of the interaction between the two therapeutic participants. This part of the interaction is thought to be an inevitable by-product of the frequent, regular contact between patient and therapist. In itself, the real relationship has received the least study or interest from psychodynamic clinicians. When it is discussed in the literature, most frequently it is mentioned in a somewhat negative way, as something to be tolerated or accepted in order for the therapeutic work to proceed.

The therapeutic alliance has been described by many dynamic writers as the working, task-oriented bond that develops between the rational, investigative, and psychologically observant aspects of the personalities of patient and therapist. Out of the alliance comes the analytic process, which includes on the part of the patient the freedom to communicate fully about inner experience and an openness to the interpretations that are offered by the therapist.

Transference and *countertransference* refer to the historically determined, irrational, idiosyncratic perceptions, affects, and portrayals
of the therapist by the patient (transference) and of the patient by
the therapist (countertransference). Transference and countertransference are generally described as an unconscious process in and
through which one participant mistakes or actively transforms the
other into someone from the former person's past. This distortion usually reflects both plausible and implausible aspects of the interaction
(Gill, 1982). Transference and countertransference bring past, internalized relationships with significant others into the immediate interaction in a repetitive and initially unacknowledged way, and they
are among the most frequent causes of resistance and blockage in the
flow of the communication between patient and therapist.

There is a deep and highly significant division in the psychoanalytic world with regard to the therapeutic utility of the therapeutic
interaction and of transference and countertransference. This division
is a consequence of a more basic psychoanalytic debate about the
nature of psychopathology. More traditional analysts, who remain
closer to a Freudian model, retain the emphasis on unconscious conflict and its resolution through insight. On the other side of the debate
are those analysts who understand psychopathology to be the manifestation of developmental deficits that are retained in faulty psychological structures. This group argues that these deficits are enacted
in the therapeutic interaction and must be repaired through novel
experiences with the therapist.

In the conflict model, the therapeutic alliance serves as the plat-
form on which free association and interpretation are built. The patient attempts to fulfil his or her assignment: to report all thoughts,
images, and experiences as freely and completely as possible. It is
the therapist's job to listen with "freely hovering attention" and to
offer interpretations of the implicit meanings of the patient's verbal
productions. As the pair move through this work, the therapist becomes part of the patient's intrapsychic life, with the result that ar-
chaic modes and patterns of representation will emerge to color the
patient's perception of the therapist. The emergence of such transference phenomena is thought to complicate and to interfere with the
alliance and with free association. As a result, the transference reactions become the focus of intensive analytic inquiry and interpretation. Countertransference reactions also emerge as old introjects and
self-images are evoked in the therapist. Most often, these reactions
are managed by a silent process of self-analysis by the therapist. Currently, a consensus has emerged that countertransference reactions

provide extremely important data about the patient's history and immediate psychodynamic situation. In fact, there is a group of psychoanalysts who advocate the judicious revelation by the therapist of such reactions (e.g., Wolstein, 1990).

Within the deficit model of psychopathology, we find analysts who argue for the primacy of interactions that are closely akin to the corrective emotional experience (Alexander & French, 1946) discussed in Chapter 3. This group has been described as advocating one or another version of the "relational" perspective within analysis (Greenberg & Mitchell, 1983) and includes followers of self psychology (Kohut, 1980), object relations theory (Winnicott, 1971), and interpersonal psychoanalysis (Levenson, 1983). In these therapies, the verbal interchange is secondary to, or is subsumed under, the powerful interpersonal exchange. The patient enacts with the therapist the ways in which he or she was neglected, traumatized, or failed by parents and others. The ability of the therapist to understand these hurts, to communicate about them effectively, and to provide the necessary curative experiences that the patient has always needed are expected to eventuate in repaired psychic structures, in new introjections and identifications, and in a revision of representations of the self and of others. New, ameliorative interpersonal experience becomes the raw material of slowly built intrapsychic repairs and configurations.

The differentiation of the interaction into "real," alliance, and transference components is downplayed in the relational deficit perspective. Instead, in one form or another, these analysts choose to emphasize issues of enactment, repetition, and participation that are closely related to the cyclical concepts contained in many integrative theories (see Chapter 2).

Among humanistic and experiential therapists, those with a client-centered orientation have made the most substantial contributions to our understanding of the therapeutic relationship. As has been stated many times, for Rogers (1957, 1961) and his followers the therapeutic interaction provided the "necessary and sufficient" conditions for change and growth. Those relationship conditions include the provision by the therapist of an utterly safe and accepting atmosphere, in which the client is responded to with unconditional positive regard or prizing, warmth, and accurate empathy. These conditions can be offered only if the therapist functions out of the experience of being as fully integrated or self-congruent as he or she can be. Any significant shift away from self-congruence by the therapist is likely to result in anxiety that will interfere with the therapist's ability to respond to the patient in an nonevaluative and open way.

The relationship conditions in this therapy allow the patient to gradually broaden and deepen his or her ability to live in feelings and experiences, and to consciously symbolize that experience to the fullest degree possible. The reason is that internalized "conditions of worth" (Rogers, 1957) that were instilled in early family life can be unlearned actively in the interaction with the therapist (Bohart, 1990). As the patient finds unconditional acceptance regardless of the nature of his or her ongoing internal experiences, he or she learns to prize, accept, and symbolize those experiences as well. The final result of this process is self-congruence and a greatly expanded potential for phenomenological authenticity on the part of the patient.

Client-centered therapy is a process-oriented therapy in which the relationship and technique are considered fully identical and inseparable (Rice & Greenberg, 1992). The "real," forward-looking, and growth-oriented aspects of the relationship are considered indispensable, to the exclusion of any meaningful consideration of regressive or transferential components or distortions of the interaction. In fact, as Shlein (1984) and other modern client-centered theorists have pointed out, in this orientation the notion of transference may have more to do with the anxieties and fears of the therapist than with any clinically meaningful events in the therapy. Shlein argued that reliance on the concept of transference by a client-centered therapist may be a way of negating or avoiding a real but painful perception of, or appropriately negative response to, the therapist by the patient. Such defensive behavior contradicts the authentic, unconditionally accepting, and congruent attitudes that typify client-centered therapy.

Existential and Gestalt therapists do not stress the efficacy of the therapeutic interaction to the extent that client-centered therapists do, but both groups agree essentially that an authentic encounter is necessary for significant change to occur (Bugenthal & Kleiner, 1993; Rice & Greenberg, 1992). Perls (1973) discussed the therapeutic relationship in the briefest of ways, but other Gestalt authors (e.g., Yontef, 1989) have pointed out that much of the distortion of bodily experience and of psychological awareness that the patient brings to therapy is part of the interaction with the therapist. Contemporary Gestalt therapy stresses the need for an honest, open, and emotionally charged exchange between patient and therapist, in which the patient is confronted immediately with his or her ways of avoiding contact with the self and with the therapist. This respectful but potent "I–Thou" experience is considered as important as the technical experiments and exercises that marked the formal Gestalt approach (Yontef, 1969, 1989).

Unlike client-centered therapists, existential therapists do not perceive technique and relationship as equivalent. The relationship is considered the sphere in which active change processes and experiential learning are encouraged and provoked (Bugenthal, 1965). Existential writers often incorporate notions of the real relationship, the therapeutic alliance, and distortion and transference into their consideration of the therapeutic relationship (Bugenthal & Kleiner, 1993; May & Yalom, 1989). However, they differ from psychoanalysts in stressing the current motives for inauthentic and defensive behavior with the therapist, which center on the patient's existential anxieties. The therapist responds to the patient's defensive and transferential attitudes and behaviors by remaining as real and authentic as possible, the result being a powerful and unsettling clash or encounter that shakes and disables the patient's ways of avoiding choices and responsibility. The "presence" of the therapist (May & Yalom, 1989) is a critical variable in this process. It is defined as the therapist being with the patient in the most fully human, authentic, unique, and open way possible. Bugenthal and Kleiner (1993) noted that the egalitarian position of patient and therapist in existential therapy may best be described as the hiring of the therapist as a consultant by the patient. Support, acceptance, exploration, advice, and confrontation are all part of this relationship.

Cognitive-behavioral therapies are built on the explicit acknowledgment of the need for a comfortable and secure therapeutic relationship. This interaction is most often described as "collaborative empiricism" (Beck et al., 1979). This term refers to the joint venture in which therapist and patient are engaged, the focus being the correction or modification of the patient's symptoms and interpersonal problems. Early writers on behavior therapy (e.g., Eysenck, 1960) decried the positive effects of the therapeutic relationship and argued that behavior therapy's impact could be traced entirely to its techniques. However, most clinically sophisticated behaviorists abandoned this view long ago. As Goldfried and Davison (1976) pointed out, technical expertise without interpersonal skill does not result in continuance in, or cooperation with, the tasks and goals of cognitive-behavioral therapy. Fishman and Lubetkin (1983) observed that the technical aspects of behavior therapy often take up only a small percentage of the time spent in sessions, more minutes being devoted to the therapeutic provision of empathy, understanding, encouragement, support, and the generation of alternative behavioral solutions.

O'Leary and Wilson (1987) suggested that issues within the therapeutic relationship in behavior therapy could not and should not be
relegated to the junk pile of "nonspecific" factors. In their view, the
patient's expectations, the intricacies of the therapist's response to the
patient, and the repetition of deviant patterns in the therapeutic interaction were all as important in determining outcome as were ex-
perimentally derived techniques. Most recently, Goldfried (Gaston,
Goldfried, Greenberg, Horvath, Raue, & Watson, 1995; Goldfried, 1995;
Raue & Goldfried, 1994) compared the role of the therapeutic relationship in cognitive-behavioral therapy to the role of anesthesia in sur-
gery: It is absolutely necessary to enable the patient to accept and
tolerate the pain that is caused by the procedure. Goldfried (1995)
recently expanded his view of the utility of the therapeutic relationship to include the patient–therapist interaction as an important source
of *in vivo* data, about which hypotheses concerning the patient's general interpersonal functioning can be generated. He included his own
reactions to the patient and the patient's appraisals of his feelings as
useful points for cognitive and behavioral intervention.

A formal theory of the specific components of the therapeutic relationship that are most important clinically has not yet been worked
out by cognitive-behavioral therapists. A number of studies have indicated that cognitive-behavioral therapists are as adept as or more
adept than therapists of other orientations in establishing a positively
charged, warm, unconditionally accepting relationship (Gold, 1980;
Raue & Goldfried, 1994; Sweet, 1985). Also, retrospective studies of
patients' experiences in behavior therapy indicate repeatedly that
those patients found the relationship at least as important in their progress as they did the technical aspects of the treatment (Raue & Goldfried, 1994). Most writers within this orientation also argue that a
major source of resistance to or noncompliance with cognitive and
behavioral techniques derives from failures of interpersonal contact by
the therapist (Gold, 1980; Goldfried & Davison, 1976; Lazarus, 1989).

TRANSFERENCE AND COUNTERTRANSFERENCE
IN TRADITIONAL PSYCHOTHERAPIES

How patient and therapist relate to each other in idiosyncratic
modes; and how they mistake each other for significant people in
the past and present lives of each, comes under study in most forms
of psychotherapy. Psychoanalysis, of course, has made the exploration

of these phenomena perhaps the central part of its technique and its clinical theory. The analysis of the transference was first mentioned in Freud's earliest writings (Breuer & Freud, 1895; Freud, 1912). As the concept of transference evolved in classical psychoanalysis, it referred to the desires and attitudes toward, and fears and perceptions of, the patient's parents, which were that gradually focused on the analyst during the process of therapy. Transference was understood to be an unconscious distortion of the person of the therapist. He or she was experienced unconsciously as someone else, the result being regressive relatedness and an unwitting demonstration of the patient's childhood conflicts, defenses, and fixations. The gradual analysis of these manifestations of transference was and is considered crucial to intrapsychic change. As the patient becomes conscious of the wishes, fears, and representations that he or she has "hung" on the neutral and relatively anonymous analyst, those issues potentially loose their grip on the person. As a result, old conflicts may be resolved, and maladaptive object representations and self-images may be modified or abandoned.

Classical psychoanalysis regards countertransference as the equivalent of transference, except for its locus in the therapist. In this framework, the therapist's unique unconscious responses to the patient are taken to be unresolved neurotic issues that can only interfere with treatment. The therapist is thought to be in a temporarily impaired state that requires self-analysis to be resolved.

In recent years, the psychoanalytic understanding and utilization of transference and countertransference have evolved considerably. Modern psychoanalysts approach these phenomena in ways that overlap extensively with the approaches of their cognitive-behavioral and humanistic colleagues. Transference is no longer considered solely the bringing forward of aspects of past relationships into a present one. Instead, psychodynamic writers (chiefly Gill, 1982, 1994; Levenson, 1983; Mitchell, 1993) have taken up ideas from constructivism, phenomenology, and hermeneutics and have evolved a conception of transference that stresses the unique blend of past and present that it represents. In these conceptions of transference, the patient's reactions to the therapist are considered plausible, creative, and potentially healthy events that transcend mere repetitions of past relationships. Also, these writers believe that each manifestation of transference contains within it some kernel of accuracy and reality with regard to the therapist's behavior, emotions, and ideas. That is, the patient's reactions may be biased by experiences and structures that are derived from past attachment but also involve an attempt to integrate and make sense of the therapist's input and involvement. As Gill (1982, 1994) has pointed out, transference reaction do not exist in a potential, latent state, just waiting to unfold. These reactions are constructed as the patient tries to grasp the meaning of her or his involvement with the therapist. And as he and others (particularly Mitchell, 1993; Wolstein, 1990) have pointed out further, the idea of transference as a distortion misses the forward-looking, often accurate aspects of the patients' involvement with the analyst.

Current psychodynamic thinking about countertransference has also undergone a major transformation. The therapist's responses to the patient are now usually seen as inevitable, and as uniquely important sources of data about the patient's psychodynamics and representational world (Kernberg, 1975; Levenson, 1983; Racker, 1968; Wolstein, 1990). In these perspectives, transference and countertransference are understood to be part of the ongoing matrix of subjective sharing of experience and of the construction of meaning that typify the analytic process. As a result, the analyst can neither avoid nor analyze away these experiences. Instead, he or she must accept, explore, and perhaps even communicate them to the patient in order to expand the mutual understanding of the experience.

Transference and countertransference are shunned as concepts and technical foci by most Rogerian therapists because of their bias against interpretation and imposition of the therapist's realities and meanings on the patient. In fact, some client-centered therapists (Shlein, 1984) have suggested that these concepts are used in the service of avoidance by therapists, who do not wish to be transparent to the patient or to look fully at their contribution, positive or negative, to the process of therapy. Implicitly, however, client-centered therapy includes the understanding that the patient's enduring modes of seeking conditional regard, and of clouding awareness, are demonstrated in relation to the therapist. This "transference" is not met with interpretation or exploration, as in dynamic therapy. As the client-centered therapist empathizes, reflects back some version of the meanings and experiences that the patient has not symbolized fully, and prizes the patient, the relationship gradually shifts toward a genuine, novel, and creatively open interchange.

While client-centered therapists do not usually refer to "countertransference," they have always made use of the feelings, thoughts, and other reactions that are evoked by the patient. In fact, these data are often the central source of the therapist's comments to the patient. The Rogerian concern (Rogers, 1957) with the therapist's ability to provide unconditional positive regard, to empathize, and to be genuine is similar to the psychodynamic view of the distorting effects of countertransference. A client-centered therapist who observed herself or himself failing to react in these ways would probably engage in much self-searching to correct the situation.

Existential therapists (Bugenthal & Kleiner, 1993; May & Yalom, 1989) often rely on notions of transference and countertransference that are very similar to psychoanalytic ideas. However, this group of therapists sees the source of these phenomena as existential anxiety and the retreat from the pain of an authentic existence. The patient reacts to the therapist as he or she does and did to others when threatened. Gradually, these transference reactions are confronted and interpreted, and a more authentic expression of self in the therapeutic exchange may emerge. Countertransference is considered the therapist's flight from authenticity (Bugenthal, 1981). The therapist who is open to the encounter is free of old patterns of engagement and relatedness.

Gestalt therapy considers transference an avoidance of the true encounter with the self and with the other (Simkin & Yontef, 1984). The patient approaches the therapist within the limits of relatedness that were learned in the past as a way of avoiding anxiety. These transference reactions are confronted and worked with actively so that the patient is assisted to more open to his or her full experience of the therapist. Gestalt therapists use their emotional reactions and openly acknowledge them to the patient. As in client-centered and existential therapies, countertransference as a label would probably be reserved for those instances in which the therapist is avoiding an authentic encounter or has place some limits on his or her awareness.

Transference and countertransference are not usually included in the writings of cognitive and behavioral psychotherapists. Earlier in the history of these approaches, this omission probably reflected the strong, open antipsychoanalytic bias of pioneers in this field, as much as or more than a lack of clinical and empirical utility of the concepts. At this point, while the terms *transference* and *countertransference* do not appear often in this literature, there are many references to similar phenomena and ideas, especially by those cognitive behaviorists who have adopted a more interpersonally oriented, process focus (e.g., Goldfried & Davison, 1976; Kanfer & Schefft, 1988; Safran & Segal, 1990). These authors observe that preexisting patterns of construing experience, of experiencing and expressing affect, and of interacting with others often emerge in the relationship with the therapist. As in most psychodynamic approaches, these manifestations of transference are believed both to block forward progress and to represent data that can be worked with immediately and effectively. Transference reactions may be tested cognitively; reduced or countered by the use of anxiety-reducing methods, behavior rehearsal, or social skills training; and then used as a source of modifying the patient's ways of thinking and behaving in a larger social circle. Most modern cognitive-behavioral theories do not expect transference to be part of the central change processes in every case, but they do work with it effectively when it does occur to a significant enough degree to interfere with other therapeutic activities (Kanfer & Schefft, 1988; Raue & Goldfried, 1994).

There is some recent acknowledgment of the presence of transference issues and distortions that may interfere with collaborative empiricism (Raue & Goldfried, 1994). These issues are generally assumed to stay in the background of the treatment process and to have little impact on outcome. This assumption stems from the idea that the continuous task focus and overt review of the collaborative aspects of the therapy keep repressive and idiosyncratic interpersonal meanings dormant. There are, however, a couple of exceptions to this position. For example Linehan's (1993; Heard & Linehan, 1994) dialectical behavior therapy of borderline personality disorder emphasizes the importance of validation by the therapist, and of acceptance and support within the therapeutic relationship. These interpersonal variables are assumed to anticipate, forestall, and correct the distortions of the therapeutic relationship that can be so destructive to the treatment of borderline patients. In the functional analytic therapy developed by Kohlenberg and Tsai (1994), a Skinnerian behavior-analytic approach includes a heavy emphasis on the patient–therapist exchange, and particularly on the manifestations of the patient's problematic functioning in the here and now. These authors noted explicitly the overlap between their model and modes of intervening and the psychodynamic approach to transference. Both of these therapies, however, are more accurately integrative in nature than they are strict versions of behavior therapy.

Countertransference is a topic rarely discussed in these approaches. Part of the reason is that cognitive-behavioral theories do not either encourage or inhibit the therapist with regard to using his or her reactions to the patient. Also, the learning theory bases of the earlier behavioral models could not easily accommodate these data. At present, a few cognitive therapists, particularly Guidano and Liotti (1983) and Safran and Segal (1990), have moved the use of the therapist's reactions to the patient into the center of the treatment process. These authors have suggested that the therapist can work most effectively to change deeper schemas and constructions if the interpersonal interactions that reinforce those ways of thinking are also changed. To make these changes, the therapist must often use his or her observations of his or her interaction with the patient, and of his or her contribution to the patient's experience, as primary sources of data. This interpersonal challenge, called "unhooking" by Safran and Segal (1990), moves cognitive therapy to a deeper level of intervention that greatly resembles some versions of interpersonal psychoanalysis (Levenson, 1983) and many psychodynamically influenced integrative therapies.

RESISTANCE IN TRADITIONAL THERAPIES

The concept of resistance originated in Freud's (1909) psychoanalytic studies and has been of central clinical and theoretical concern in psychoanalysis since that time. Originally seen as a phenomenon that was antithetical to the process of treatment, resistance has long been redefined as an inevitable, necessary, and positive part of dynamic work.

Resistance refers both to gross behavioral acts of omission and commission, such as refusing to talk to the therapist or missing an appointment, and to more subtle actions and intrapsychic processes. These latter are more subjective than the former and involve encroachment on the patient's associations of his or her characteristic defense mechanisms and personality traits. Thus, resistance may be understood as a process of distortion, avoidance, or flight when sensitive material is close to the patient's consciousness. This material violates the patient's standards of safety, social acceptability, or personal integrity and therefore provokes anxiety, shame, guilt, or some other dysphoria. These affects call out unwitting and powerful efforts to limit what material may enter consciousness; these efforts are considered resistance when observed in a clinical situation.

The entire process that was just described may occur at any level of consciousness; however, "true" resistance in the psychoanalytic sense is largely an unconscious process. The self-monitoring, reactive affects, defensive reactions, and underlying fantasies, desires, or feelings are knowable only indirectly to patient and therapist. Resistance makes itself known in the content of the patient's report, and in his or her style of speaking. Resistant activity is signaled by gaps in the patient's associations; by subtle or abrupt shifts in content and in the direction of thought; by momentary forgetting, slips, or confusion; and by an exaggeration or diminution of the affect associated with some verbal matter.

Resistance signals the *in vivo* activation of some intrapsychic conflict in the here and now of the therapeutic interaction. As a result, the awareness by the therapist of resistance is usually the starting point of psychodynamic interpretive work. Interpretations often begin with the therapist calling the patient's attention to a change, gap, or block in the associative process. Once this can be seen by the patient, it is explored motivationally and in terms of the affects and defenses that were employed; the full interpretation of resistance requires the understanding of what material the patient sought to keep out of awareness, the meaning of that material should it become conscious, the effects on the patient and the therapist that were to be avoided, and the specific dysphoria that prompted the process.

Interpretations of resistance are rarely successful the first time that they are offered, as this is a tenacious process. Singer (1965) pointed out that resistance in psychotherapy is a remnant of the patient's earliest and most pervasive survival strategies and suggested that the person learned these reactions while growing up in order to manage and control emotional dangers in the most important interpersonal relationships. For example, if the child learned to fear being angry and to repress that emotion in order to balance a relationship with a parent who would not tolerate that emotion in the child, then repression of anger may occur in many significant relationships when that child becomes an adult, including, of course, the relationship with the therapist.

The perspective of resistance serving an outmoded survival function pervades most psychodynamic thinking today, sometimes overtly, and often in an unacknowledged way. Analysis of these patterns of organizing relationships and of protecting oneself and others from the contents of the mind has been the framework of psychoanalytic technique since Reich's (1949) book on character analysis. In many psychoanalytic therapies, it occupies a large majority of the time spent by therapist and patient. As resistance is understood, it can be altered, resolved, or given up by the patient, who finds survival to be less tenuous than he or she perceived it to be as a child. The anxiety, guilt, shame, and other affects associated with certain motives or fantasies are lessened, the result being increased self-awareness and psychological integration.

Client-centered therapy does not often refer to ideas about resistance or noncompliant behavior. However, in Rogers's (1961) clinical discussions, resistance can be inferred to occur when anxiety causes the client to distort his or her experience, and therefore to present himself or herself in ungenuine, incongruent ways. Essentially, Gestalt therapy and existential therapy share this viewpoint, in portraying resistance as an in-therapy enactment of the ways in which the patient avoids a true, authentic expression of feelings and experience. Such in authenticity is met with active confrontation, exploration, and examination in Gestalt and existential work. In the Rogerian tradition, the processes of avoidance or distortion are dealt with indirectly. The therapist's gentle refusal to respond to ungenuine experience, as well as the reflection of the underlying meanings and experiences, gradually allows the person to let go of such defensive states.

Client-centered therapists differ considerably from existential and Gestalt therapists in the consideration and therapeutic use of resistance. In fact the term itself rarely, if ever, appears in the client-centered literature. Such a concept is theoretically and clinically antithetical to the Rogerian emphasis on unconditional prizing and acceptance of the patient. In order to incorporate the idea of resistance into client-centered therapy, the therapist would also have to assume a stance in which he or she supposes greater knowledge about the patient's experience and behavior than the patient has at that moment. This kind of assumption cannot be fit easily into the framework of client-centered work.

Shlein (1984) argued cogently that concepts such as resistance are more reflective of the therapist's inability to understand and to empathize with the patient than of aspects of the patient's psychology. He equated the labeling of a patient's puzzling or unpleasant behavior as resistance as the therapist's efforts to avoid his or her input into those actions. For example, when the patient is uncooperative or is anxiously avoiding listening to the therapist, it behooves the therapist to consider how he or she has failed, hurt, or frightened the patient, rather than to look for an explanation based on the client's conflicts and history. Most client-centered therapists would agree to the observation that the patient often behaves and communicates in an anxiety-driven manner, in which he or she is more concern about the therapist's reactions and experiences than about his or her own. At these times the patient seems to be more interested in provoking the therapist or obtaining a response from the therapist, and/or in avoiding some aspect of the patient's experiences of which he or she is only dimly aware. These experiences reflect the influence of the patient's childhood learning experiences, in which aspects of the self were not prized and accepted by parents and other adults. However, these moments in therapy are not distinguished by a change in technique on the part of the therapist. As the therapist attempts to understand the patient's anxiety and distortions of awareness in the ongoing atmosphere of empathy, unconditional positive regard, and openness, the patient may be able to recognize and to overcome his or her distortions and avoidances without other intervention.

Gestalt therapists and existential therapists share a more active and confrontational style in working with patient resistances. Both groups are concerned primarily with pointing out to the patient the ways in which he or she avoids certain experiences, self-knowledge, and affective states. Unlike for psychodynamic therapists, the "why's," or motivational conflicts that cause resistance, are of less importance than the "how's," that is, the ways in which the patient becomes or remains in authentic or blocked with regard to important bodily and psychological sensations and desires. Gestalt therapists (e.g., Perls, Goodman, & Hefferline, 1951) have suggested that blockages in awareness are manifestations of internalized parental and social prohibitions against certain types of pleasure, desire, or awarenesses. In the existential tradition (e.g., Bugenthal & Kleiner, 1993; May & Yalom, 1989), resistance follows from the dim perception of some type of existential anxiety, for example, the fearsome awareness of death, limits, or the other aspects of "thrownness." Central to both schools of therapy are the therapist's steadfast confrontation of the patient's lack of cooperation with exercises (in Gestalt therapy) and the patient's attempts to win favor with or to create distance from the therapist, or to avoid painful situations and experiences.

Most discussions of resistance in the cognitive-behavioral literature are concerned with the breakdown of the collaborative exchange between patient and therapist. In this perspective, resistance is often renamed *noncompliance*. Noncompliant behavior takes the form of a patient's failing to understand or to complete homework assignments, changing the topic that is being discussed in therapy sessions, or straying from an agreed-upon agenda for a particular therapeutic sequence.

Unlike dynamic or humanistic therapies, which locate the origins of resistance within the psychology of the patient, cognitive-behavioral therapies stress the input and role of the therapist in causing noncompliance (Beck et al., 1979; Lazarus, 1989; Wachtel, 1985). These authors have argued that therapist error and lack of interpersonal skill are the most frequent and important reasons why patients cease to cooperate with therapeutic plans and procedures. Chief among these errors are inaccurate understanding and formulations of

the patient's problems and goals, which then lead to technical suggestions that are distasteful, useless, or incomprehensible to the patient. An intervention that is not perceived to address the patient's
most pressing fears or discomforts is less likely to be adhered to by
the patient than is one that conveys the therapist's willingness and
ability to be helpful. The failure by the therapist to fully explain the
rationale, methods, effects, and discomforts of any technique is also
implicated in limited compliance.

Finally, a lack of respect of and of individualized concern for
the patient, the failure to ask the patient about his or her thoughts
and feelings on interventions and suggestions, the therapist's general
difficulty in being open to feedback and to true collaboration have
also been implicated in patient noncompliance.

A few investigators have sought to identify patient-generated
sources of resistance or noncompliance in cognitive-behavioral therapies. An early and highly significant paper concerned with the topic
was published by Davison (1973), who equated resistance with efforts
at "countercontrol" by the patient. This term and concept refer to the
power differential that is inherently part of the relationship between
patient and therapist in any form of therapy. For individuals who
have been sensitized to rebel against authority early in life, the directive expertise of the cognitive-behavioral therapist may be intoler-
able. Such patients feel compelled to fight the therapist's efforts,
either covertly or overtly ways. What emerges is an interaction in
which the patient's perceptions of having the upper hand, of being
in control of the situation or of the therapist, becomes more important
than the alleviation of his or her complaints and symptoms. Gold
(1980) found that many of the intrapsychic sources of resistance identified by psychoanalysts are also influential in cognitive-behavioral
therapy. Patients attributed noncompliance to both overly strong positive and negative feelings about their therapists, to preexisting conflicts, to anxiety generated by the techniques, and to a general need
to avoid interpersonal contact.

The interpersonal attitude that underlies efforts at countercontrol
has been termed *reactance* and has been found to be a frequent and
powerful impediment to success in straightforward cognitive-behavioral approaches (Dowd, 1994). Other sources of resistance that arise
in the patient's psychology seem to resemble the variables that are
stressed in the psychoanalytic literature: anxiety and conflict about
change; avoidance of painful situations, affects, memories, or images
of self and others; and powerful negative and positive reactions to
the therapist and his or her techniques (Gold, 1980). In this last cate-

gory are such experiences as feeling rejected, disliked, or misunderstood by the therapist; feeling sexually attracted to the therapist; or being in awe of the therapist and feeling needy, shamed, or guilty in his or her presence. These perceptions and emotions greatly resemble descriptions of transference in dynamic psychotherapy and are correlated with high levels of noncompliance (Gold, 1980).

INTEGRATIVE APPROACHES TO THE PSYCHOTHERAPEUTIC INTERACTION

Lacking a universally accepted framework for discussion of the therapeutic interaction, I now propose and will utilize below three facets of the interaction between patient and therapist that can be examined and compared in a cross-sectional basis: the *emotional climate* of the interaction, the *interactional stance,* and the *role of interactional data.*

The Emotional Climate of the Therapeutic Interaction

The emotional climate refers to the quality and quantity of affective engagement and involvement between patient and therapist that are thought to be helpful, necessary, or ameliorative. Also important here are the specific types of affective and interpersonal experiences that are deemed to be positive, neutral, or destructive in the therapeutic work.

As a group, integrative therapists seem to be in broad consensus with each other, and with modern trends in the sectarian schools of psychotherapy, which emphasize the need for, and the importance of, a warm, respectful, and empathic approach to the patient. Their opinions would not be met by much disagreement from many psychoanalysts, cognitive-behavioral therapists, or humanistic therapists. In the analytic community, as noted above, there has been a significant trend toward an acknowledgment of the central role of warmth and empathy (Kohut, 1977), the provision of a comforting, protective "holding" environment (Winnicott, 1971), and the need for a sense of safety, security, and freedom from excessive anxiety in the therapeutic setting (Sandler, 1960; Sullivan, 1953). Cognitive-behavioral therapy, as represented by Beck (1976) and Goldfried and Davison (1976), has emphasized these emotional components as well, as have humanistic therapists since that form of therapy was introduced (see Rogers, 1957).

An accepting, safe, and empathic emotional climate is considered necessary to allow the patient to reveal his or her intrapsychic and behavior difficulties, and the attachment and closeness that grow out of warmth and empathy are viewed by most writers as two of the bases of behavioral experimentation and cognitive, emotional, and motivational revelation and change.

For the majority of integrative therapists, this emotional climate of empathy and acceptance provides the patient with a new sense of self-worth, confirmation, self-acceptance and is a significant ingredient in the disconfirmation of old and dysfunctional thoughts, opinions, and feelings about the self and others. This position is exemplified by the work of Andrews (1993), Wachtel (1993; Gold & Wachtel, 1993), and Greenberg et al. (1993), all of whom have pointed out the need for safety, closeness, and confirmation of the patient within the therapy before confrontation, challenges, and change can occur. Similarly, in discussions of integrative therapy with substance abusers and with chronic pain patients respectively, Cummings (1993) and Dworkin and Grzesiak (1993) have emphasized early bonding and the siding of therapist with patient as necessary steps in the early stages of treatment. Allen's (1993) unified systems approach also begins with such efforts at building a safe climate for bonding, which can serve as a springboard for further work. As a final example, Becker's (1993) work with organically impaired patients relied heavily on monitoring and repairing the damage to the positive bond between patient and therapist that was caused by exploration of the humiliation and shame attendant on neurological dysfunction.

Several integrative efforts, including those by Gold (1993a), Hayes and Newman (1993), and Papouchis and Passman (1993), have emphasized the role of early attachment experiences in the etiology of psychopathology and have included some stress how pathogenic beliefs and feelings about attachment can be tested and discarded on the basis of a positive and successful experience of relatedness to and with the therapist. This view, which approximates the corrective emotional experience identified by Alexander and French (1946), or the "necessary-and-sufficient" theory of the therapeutic relationship offered is shared by almost all integrative contributors to one degree or another, though none would suggest that the emotional climate by itself is totally and completely responsible for therapeutic change. Most would argue that empathic engagement is indeed necessary but is not sufficient to produce much meaningful change in and of itself. In the view of Allen (1993), Andrews (1993), Beutler and Hodgson (1993), Cummings (1993), Fodor (1993), Gold and Wachtel (1993), and

Reeve et al. (1993), among many others, this climate of empathy and safety allows the therapist to be heard when he or she challenges the patient to change an idea, behavior, or self-image, and it permits and encourages the patient to face distasteful, fearsome, or painful inner states, interpersonal events, or new behavioral challenges.

Interactional Stance

The interactional stance in the therapeutic interaction is defined in terms of such issues as the therapist's activity level; the roles and responsibilities assigned to both patient and therapist; and the place of the specific therapy on such continua as egalitarian versus authoritarian, directive versus nondirective, and exploratory versus didactic. Once again, a surprising level of consensus exists among the integrative therapists, as a group, who are cited in this book. The large majority have defined their role as encompassing both didactic and exploratory dimensions, with freedom of movement between both. There exists much agreement about and a great emphasis on the necessity and complementary nature of periods of directive teaching with moments and long expanses of exploration, while the therapist facilitates by nondirective means. Crass authoritarian attitudes and behaviors are nowhere to be found, and the didactic and directive activities of the therapists are typically presented as best set within a context of collaboration and an egalitarian approach to hypothesis testing. As described by Bugenthal and Kleiner (1993), the therapist may best take the role of a consultant who assists through his or her expertise and authority, rather than dictates or controls. The patient most frequently is considered the final arbiter of the validity and utility of the therapist's suggestions and interventions.

The role definitions provided by many integrative writers for the therapist are thus multidimensional and synthesize various sectarian positions. The therapist is understood to be a potential model, to be a source of new information about the self and the world, and to be someone whose actions stimulate new ideas, feelings, and wishes as well as confirm or disconfirm old experiences and inner states. Moderate to high levels of engagement and activity, at points or throughout the therapy, are prescribed and encouraged. These therapists do not endorse the sanctions against personal influence and guidance shared by classical psychoanalysis or by some versions of client-centered and other humanistic therapies. Anonymity, neutrality, and unconditional positive regard are considered impossibilities that even if achievable, would not fit into or make therapeutic sense in the context of the theories and methods of many, if not most, integrative positions.

This consensual stance most resembles the active "collaborative empiricism" described by Beck (1976) and the directed-inquiry method favored by Sullivan (1953) in his interpersonal psychotherapy, and therefore, it does not come as a surprise that these therapies and their methods are heavily cited as influential, especially by those writers whose work draws in other significant ways on the psychodynamic and humanistic traditions. The relative inactivity and striving for a stance in which the therapist neither teaches nor influences have been understood to be unfortunate and to be among the least helpful aspects of these solitary therapies. As Becker (1993), Gold and Wachtel (1993), Gold and Stricker (1993), Papouchis and Passman (1993), and many others have pointed out, it was these considerations that, to a great extent, encouraged integration in the first place.

The patient's role in the therapy is also understood in highly similar ways by the various authors cited. In an egalitarian, collaborative, and active therapy, the patient is considered an intelligent, educable, and vigorous participant. Most work in psychotherapy integration stresses, or implicitly regards, "role induction" (Luborsky, 1984) as an extremely important activity. Instruction in the roles and behavior associated with patienthood may be critical in helping the patient be clear about what her or she is expected to do and how the therapist will behave and how the therapy will progress, and especially in comprehending the ways in which the patient may help her or his own therapy along. Many integrative therapies have incorporated the cognitive-behavioral and systems methods of homework assignments, *in vivo* exercises, and environmental manipulation by therapist and patient, thus extending and redefining the role of both parties and their interpersonal stance toward and with each other. In almost all cases, the patient is expected to evaluate and to respond to the therapist's interventions and actions on the basis of the patient's successes and failures and emotional, cognitive, imaginative, and systemic experiences and is taught to expect a respectful and open reaction to such feedback by the therapist. As examples of this emphasis on activity and responsibility on the part of the patient, the contributions of Bugenthal and Kleiner (1993), Cummings (1993), and Ryle and Low (1993) may be cited. Here are three theories and methods that differ greatly in content and form; yet all three explicitly argue that success in treatment depends in large part on the extent to which the patient can take on, or can be moved to accept, an invested, motivated, and responsible role.

The Role of Interactional Data

Mention of the importance and utility of interactional data in psychotherapy integration is almost ubiquitous. Without exception, a strong and stable therapeutic alliance is deemed critical to ongoing therapeutic activity, and disruptions in the bond, or an inability to form such a bond, inevitably become the focus of much therapeutic concern and activity in all of the therapies under review.

Certain integrative therapists, most notably Becker (1993), Cummings (1993), Dworkin and Grzesiak (1993), Fitzpatrick (1993), Franklin, Carter, and Grace (1993), and Sollod (1993), do not venture in detail far beyond such notation of the impact of the therapeutic alliance, and their views on the use of interactional data must be inferred from their general positions on the processes of therapy. These inferences dovetail considerably with the trends that emerge from reviewing the more developed and specific approaches to interactional data in the other chapters. Three strong and related ways of conceptualizing and working with interactional data seem to be present and may be labeled the *intrapsychic-tranferential mode,* the *interpersonal-characterological mode,* and the *prizing-safety mode.*

Writers who belong to the intrapsychic-transferential mode typically see the interaction as determined by internalized needs, wishes, conflicts, defenses, and self- and object representations. The ongoing present relationship with the therapist is therefore colored by some degree of regression, distortion, and resistance to intimacy and self-disclosure. Of critical weight in this mode is the primary assumption that internal and past experience is re-created and relived, and secondary significance is attached to the unique characteristics and behavior of the therapist. This mode is nearly identical to classical and contemporary models of psychoanalysis and is most influential in the work of those integrative therapists who have incorporated ideas from a formal, intrapsychic psychodynamic model, like Bugenthal and Kleiner (1993), Fensterheim (1993), Healy (1993), Hellcamp (1993), Papouchis and Passman (1993), Rubin (1993), and Ryle and Low (1993). An intrapsychic conceptualization of interactional data orients the therapy toward certain interventive decisions and techniques. Interpretations of unconscious distortions, either as a silent guide to the therapist or out loud to the patient, are seen as critical, though interventions from other schools may be used once the transference is formulated. Anxiety and resistance are primarily understood to be intrapsychically generated and to be a result of past experience, and they are worked with accordingly.

The interpersonal-characterological mode of understanding and dealing with interactional phenomena is typical of the efforts at integration that are more indebted to interpersonal theories and psychotherapies, such as those of Sullivan (1953), and to contemporary systemic and cognitive-behavioral models and methods than to strictly psychoanalytic constructs. This mode is predominant in the ideas of Allen (1993), Andrews (1993), Beutler and Hodgson (1993), Fodor (1993), Gold (1993b), Gold and Wachtel (1993), Hayes and Newman (1993), Reeve et al. (1993), Kirschner and Kirschner (1993), and Westerman (1993), and it broadens the understanding of the interaction to include the idea that patient and therapist are mutually influencing and that the data of their interaction are often a unique blend of the past and the present.

In this mode, the therapeutic interaction is construed as embodying *in vivo* the patient's characteristic ways of engaging other people, and as both expressing and avoiding inner states. Most critically, how the patient re-creates the past and therefore maintains and reinforces his or her psychopathology by shaping other people to enter into interactions that confirm and reinforce pathogenic ideas, wishes, feelings, and representations is understood to shape and to be inevitable within the therapeutic interaction. Such patterns of confirmation (Andrews, 1993), vicious circles and the creation of accomplices (Gold & Wachtel, 1993; Wachtel, 1977), or hooking (Reeve et al., 1993) are also known by other names but are the central construct in all of the chapters that fall within this mode. Technically, this shared understanding of the interaction leads to a consensus about the need for confrontation of such patterns, an examination of how both parties have colluded in this re-creation, and in-session and out-of-session experiences aimed at breaking the hold of the characterological issues and structures that keep these patterns alive.

The interpersonal-characterological approach contains within it implicit or explicit pressures on the therapist to act within the relationship in ways that inhibit old patterns from coalescing and that appeal for fresh, novel, and risky new ways of relatedness. In some ways, technique and relationship are more fully blended in this mode than in the alternate intrapsychic mode, which comes closer to the older tradition of talking about relatedness and the need for change, rather than relating in ways meant to produce change.

This mode suggests that anxieties and resistances may be as frequently caused by interactional factors as by variables that are internal to the patient. This view calls on the therapist, then, to review the interaction and his or her own participation in order to discover any interactional sources of resistance, which if found must be met by behavioral and attitudinal changes on the therapist's part. Fensterheim (1993) cited an example of a therapy that was stalled by the therapist's fear of the patient's aggression, and that moved to a successful conclusion only after the therapist was desensitized to that experience and was able to comfortably allow the patient to be angry in sessions. Westerman (1993) argued that patient and therapist are interdependent actors who cannot help but influence each other in growth-promoting or pathogenic ways. Such a conceptualization places much greater and more explicit technical emphasis on the therapist's experiences of, and reaction to, the patient than does the intrapsychic mode, in which such reactions are handled more traditionally as countertransference.

There is no mention in any integrative writings of rigid strictures or prohibitions on utilizing the subjective experience of the therapist as a source of potential knowledge about the patient. Several writers, including Healy (1993), Reeve et al. (1993), and Sollod (1993), have explicitly advocated the need for an intensive and extensive inward focus at central points in the therapy. However, within the two modes of approaching the interaction, certain distinctions are notable how these experiences influence further process. While writers in the intrapsychic-transference mode do not object to judicious self-disclosure, and some (e.g., Bugenthal & Kleiner, 1993; Healy, 1993; Rubin, 1993) have explicitly advocated self-disclosure, such action on the part of the therapist is not fully integrated into the technical framework of treatment. That is, the role of revelation by the therapist cannot be linked to a particular goal *a priori,* and instead, such information is usually offered for spontaneous and somewhat idiosyncratic reasons.

In the interpersonal-characterological mode, therapist self-examination and interventions drawn from such scrutiny (what Reeve et al., 1993, called the therapist's "discipline") are more fully integrated into the conceptual and technical models of the therapeutic process. When the therapist offers the patient a glimpse of the therapist's experience of the patient, this information becomes the starting point for work within the hooking, vicious circles, or characterological patterns of avoidance and confirmation that typify the patient's general life situation. Similarly, while it is doubtful that any integrative therapist would argue against the importance of modeling and vicarious learning within therapy, writers in the interpersonal-characterological mode have tended to stress this aspect of the interaction. For example, Fodor (1993) suggested that the therapist's experiences in problem solving and in empowering herself or himself can be told to the patient in order to open up new possibilities of thought and behavior. Gold and Stricker (1993) suggested that the therapist encourage new internal structures through corrective and informative involvement of patient and therapist, while Gold and Wachtel (1993) pointed out that answering questions, giving advice, and sharing reactions and ideas may help the patient to end his or her involvement in repetitive and redundant negative relationships with others who refuse to be helpful.

Regression within the therapeutic interaction is acknowledged as a real and frequent phenomenon, but it is one that is not sought after, and often, efforts are recommended to counter or undermine extreme regressive and transferential experiences. This opinion seems to be shared by therapists from both interactional modes. Allen (1993) pointed out that a therapist operating within the framework of his unified therapy would seek to inhibit or undo any sign of a transference neurosis, while other authors such as Andrews (1993), Cummings (1993), and Kirschner and Kirschner (1993) have suggested deliberate therapist behavior that will surprise the patient and that will open the patient to the differences between past and present within the interaction.

Consensually, integrative therapists appear to avoid extreme reactions within therapy sessions, believing that such upheavals will produce more interference and resistance than is helpful or necessary. Papouchis and Passman (1993), who lean toward the intrapsychic mode, suggested that, frequently, the transference cannot be acknowledged or worked with openly in work with the elderly but must be "lived" or managed silently by the therapist. In the interpersonal-characterological mode, regression is particularly avoided, as such phenomena are considered representative of a very small number of situations in the patient's life and regressive events do not convey more valuable or deeper aspects of the patients experience. Gold and Wachtel's (1993) discussion of the fallacies of the "wooly mammoth" aspects of traditional psychodynamic theory is one statement of this position. Interactional data that inform and demonstrate who the patient lives as in the here and now, with real figures in his or her life, are valued much more than artificially induced regressive experiences.

Integrative psychotherapies that are built on client-centered and experiential systems (Bohart, 1990; Greenberg et al., 1993) are examples of the *prizing-safety* mode. These systems tend to accentuate the real and alliance aspects of the psychotherapeutic relationship. These systems stress that the gradual development by therapist and patient of a shared task orientation in which experiential learning, inside and outside the therapeutic interaction, is the key component of change. An atmosphere of prizing, unconditional regard, and warmth is most likely to encourage a patient to face his or her fears and previously warded-off inner experiences. These interactional conditions are the prerequisites for the development of a collaborative alliance with the therapist (Bordin, 1994; Watson & Greenberg, 1994). Once this alliance has been established, the more technical portions of the therapy can be approached. The maintenance of a warm, prizing, and collaborative alliance is thought to maximize patient compliance with active experiential tasks and exercises, while lessening the frequency of resistance and avoidant behavior. Similarly, successful completion of tasks and exercises is probably the best way to strengthen the bond between patient and therapist. In effect, technique and relationship exist in a mutually influential feedback loop.

In concluding of this section, I want to point out that the modes that I have described above are not completely contradictory, and that, in actual practice, it is likely that therapists utilize both, while perhaps emphasizing one. The integrative approach described by Gold and Stricker (1993) actually includes something of a hybrid model, in which the intrapsychic and interpersonal are given about equal weight theoretically and practically.

Neither mode would dismiss the other completely. It is more a matter of directional emphasis, as discussed by Gold (1992), in considering whether the present interaction is a shadow of the past and is caused by distant events, or the past stays live because of current interactional experiences.

Implications

Earlier in this chapter, I mentioned that conceptions of the psychotherapeutic relationship can either shape or be shaped by any therapeutic system of process and intervention. Not a single example of the former case can be found in this book. Without exception, the construal of the interaction follows from the particular ideas about psychopathology and change that mark each chapter's approach to integration. This situation is fairly equivalent to the state of affairs in the general field of psychotherapy, sectarian or integrative. Few therapies are defined by their understanding of the therapeutic relationship; instead, technical guidelines and the theory of cure and change inform the therapist with regard to the ideal and sought-after relationship. Yet the repeated convergences among integrative therapists in their approach to and use of the interaction mirrors the new similarities between therapists of sectarian schools in both form and content.

Psychotherapy in general seems to be moving toward an the greater appreciation of its interpersonal dimension, which was first advocated by Sullivan (1953), and which was adapted and expanded by Fromm-Reichman (1950), Singer (1965), Carson (1969), and Kiesler (1982), among others. Within the integrative psychotherapy community as well as without, the interaction is consensually defined as the arena in which the patient's inner world, character, cognitions, experiences, emotions, and dynamics are displayed and the place in which his or her systemic and interpersonal strengths and weaknesses are experienced and observed *in vivo* by and with the therapist. The therapist's role of participant-observer as first described by Sullivan (1953) is equally valid and applicable today in integrative therapy. In many ways, current integrative perspectives are in accordance with Sullivan's (1953) vision of his interpersonal theory, which was perhaps an unintegrative therapy in its blending of psychoanalytic ideas with concepts drawn from sociology, social psychology, anthropology, economics, linguistics, and communications theory. This is not an idle or purely academic point. Alford and Norcross (1991) and Beck (1991) have argued that cognitive therapy be considered an, or perhaps *the,* example of a mature integrative psychotherapy. Cognitive therapy is indeed powerfully represented as a component of many integrative positions, and yet its ideas and techniques do not possess the same cross-sectional influence as the repeated interpersonal emphases that have been described above in this chapter.

My point is that a start toward a mature and fully expanded theory of the psychotherapeutic interaction may well be found in the convergences in ideas of the contributors to the integrative psychotherapy literature, and in the tenets of interpersonal psychotherapy in general. In turn, such a conceptualization of the therapeutic interaction may give rise in the future to a truly unified or *integrated* form of psychotherapy that will be, in fact, seamless (Wachtel, 1991), and that will be impervious to charges of "technical eclecticism" without a consistent and integrated theoretical base (Arkowitz & Messer, 1984). In this hypothetical psychotherapy, interventions would be determined by the state of the therapeutic interaction and by which interactional factors, in or outside the relationship, need to be addressed in order to move the patient along. A comprehensive theory of any interpersonal relationship, psychotherapeutic or otherwise, must include a discussion of psychodynamic, cognitive, emotional, experiential, behavioral, and systemic variables and must account for the multidirectional nature of the causality and influence of those variables (Gold, 1992). A theory built from the start that would include all aspects of human experience would surmount and bypass the need for integration at all.

We are far from such an ideal. Yet again, the surprising and substantial quantity of agreement within the field of psychotherapy integration suggests that at some collective level such a nascent unity may exist or at least be forming. In the next section of this chapter, the narrational model of integration is used to conceptualize the therapeutic interaction.

THE NARRATIONAL APPROACH TO THE INTEGRATIVE THERAPEUTIC RELATIONSHIP

The therapeutic relationship is the vehicle for talking about the narrative, for allowing past and present components of the narrative to be enacted and demonstrated *in vivo,* and, ultimately, for the creation of new experiences that can be used to modify the narrative in a health-promoting way.

The patient's narrative provides the shape and structure of the therapeutic relationship. The patient tells the therapist what he or she knows of the story of his or her symptoms, history, and relationships. Typically, as the therapy proceeds, the therapist is drawn into the narrative, and the processes of transference and countertransference emerge. These result initially in the therapist's being drawn into the story, and living out issues with important figures in the patient's life. As the therapist becomes aware of this participation in the narrative, he or she overtly and covertly challenges that story and the role to which he or she has been assigned. This challenge is implicit in most techniques and interactions. It results in the gradual breaking up of the hold on the patient of his or her grim, destructive narration.

During, and because of, this telling, a new subplot in the story is created as the relationship between the two participants unfolds and develops. This subplot often evolves later as the central story line around which future experiences evolve and are organized. That is, a helpful experience with the therapist can serve to "close the book" on the patient's life up to that point. New gains, more positive self-images drawn from the therapeutic interaction, and more benign images of others that derive from the patient's experiences with the therapist may populate and define the bulk of the posttherapy narrative.

Each patient comes to therapy having portrayed himself or herself as being in need of some kind of assistance. In a complementary way, the therapist is cast in the role of the helper. This broad script enables the patient to tell his or her story to the therapist, who not only listens and tries to be helpful but becomes enmeshed in the story by forming a bond with the patient. Different stories require different interpersonal approaches by the therapist, resulting in a therapeutic stance that allows for specifying and tailoring the nature of the therapeutic interaction on individualized clinical grounds, rather than *a priori* theoretical issues. In other words, some narratives are best met with neutral inquiry and interpretation of the missing elements, those elements being unconscious conflict, self- and object images, and anxieties. Other pathogenic stories respond best to didactic instruction, when the tale is one of lost or misshapen learning and thinking. A person whose narrative is marked by a lack of adaptive learning experiences and by gaps in adaptational skills will probably appreciate and join readily with an expert teacher and helper. Patients whose scripts unfold with lack of genuine access to their own experience and meanings may require an interaction marked by unconditional positive regard or by emotionally charged confrontation. For example, a patient whose life story suggests an early life in which prizing, empathy, and unconditional positive regard were absent will not flourish readily in the neutral atmosphere of psychoanalysis, or in the instructional and directive interaction promoted by cognitive-behavioral therapies. These differing relationship requirements reflect the particular aspects of each patient's narrative that contributed to the development of his or her psychopathology.

It is likely that many patients need and will greatly benefit from a therapeutic relationship in which the therapist can shift from one type of engagement to another as different issues and problems arise. As the patient's story unfolds and is examined, the unique blend of dynamic conflict, unsymbolized experience and affect, self- and object disturbances, cognitive distortions, behavioral dysfunctions, and interpersonal vicious circles will be observed, discussed, inferred, and enacted. Technical decisions will interact immediately with interactional considerations, in that the choice of any single intervention brings with it an optimal type of relationship. Interventions also bring with them different types of opportunities for modifying narratives. For example, when the therapist suggests desensitization for an anxiety symptom, he or she has structured the relationship in one

way, while confronting an in authentic engagement moves the interaction into another sphere. The new experiences that may result from
these techniques will perhaps contradict a defective part of the patient's story or may fill in a gap. These and any other technical decisions become part of the new subplot that the patient and the
therapist together are writing. The outcome of these interventions can
become the raw material for a further revision of the patient's story,
or even for a totally new characterization of the self, of others, and
of the world. So, any consideration of technique must always be
placed within the immediate and distant context of the unique relationship and plot that the dyad have developed.

The form and content of the interaction between patient and therapist will convey much of what happened in the past, as well as what
happens in the present between the patient and significant people in
his or her life. The therapist's responses to these enactments will serve
to heighten the patient's awareness of these vicious circles, and of the
parts of the narrative that they convey and contain. Eventually, the
patient will learn to anticipate them or to extricate himself or herself
from them. As important, the novelty of this kind of successful adaptation and the newly available spontaneity and creativity of the therapeutic interaction become critical sources of raw material from which
revisions and corrections of, and additions to, existing narratives can
be drawn. The experience of the therapist, of his or her efforts at helping, of prizing, teaching, interpreting, or failing honestly, becomes a
new part of the story about the self, about others, and about what is
possible, expectable, and realistically hopeful in life.

CASE EXAMPLE: JAMES

James approached psychotherapy and the therapist as he did
most other people in his life. He came in leading with his best shot:
He brought his prodigious intellectual talents and critical capacities
to bear on the very notion of the therapy as potentially helpful. Almost from the first words spoken, a debate was established in which
James argued for the naysayers and, at the same time, gave the therapist little space or time to question, rebut, or state an opposing point
of view. James was uniquely aware of the clinical and research literature, was as familiar as, or even more familiar than, the therapist
with outcome studies of both psychotherapy and pharmacotherapy,

and he made a strong case for accepting a neurochemical etiology for his psychological distress.

It would have been easy, theoretically appropriate, and probably pointless to conceptualize and interpret James's argumentative interaction as resistant or as demonstrative of reactance leading to countercontrol behaviors. However, it seemed fairly obvious that intervening in this way would have led to the incorporation of the therapist's input into the debate in a useless way. It was more than likely that James would have some data to disqualify each effort at every interpretation, cognitively oriented query, or behavioral suggestion. As important, the therapist's responses to James during this period seemed to tell a different tale from one of resistance or reactance. The therapist felt admiration for James intellectual gifts and for his skill as a devil's advocate. He did not feel devalued or demeaned; instead he experienced James's participation as an indication of the unspoken importance that the patient placed on his contact with the therapist.

The therapist began to speculate that James was in effect living out and telling interactionally a crucial piece of his narrative: that of the intellectually precocious and gifted child whose enthusiasm for the world of ideas, facts, and learning had been ignored by his parents. This historical formulation was checked with James, who acknowledged it with some surprised and apparent pain. The confirmation of this bit of the narrative led to the adoption by the therapist of an admiring, prizing stance with regard to James's intellectual quest to discredit the therapy. The therapist limited his focus to understanding how James obtained new information, to sharing his appreciation of James's fund of knowledge and extraordinary critical abilities, and to responding empathically to the patient's doubts about psychotherapy.

Here we find the demonstration of integration concepts such as hooking (Safran & Segal, 1990) or vicious circles (Gold & Wachtel, 1993). James was unfolding his narrative in the presence of the therapist. As he did so, he invited and often induced the therapist to take complementary roles that would complete and reinforce the story as it already existed. For example, James's intellectual, smug dismissal of psychotherapy could, and did, evoke feelings of detachment, anxiety, anger, and guilt in the therapist, all of which might have led him to attack James, or to withdraw from James. The former response, of course, would have confirmed James's anxieties about interpersonal contact, while the second (withdrawal) would have been an enactment of a deeper part of the story: his parents' distance and lack of involvement. Wishing to be neither type of accomplice, the therapist attempted to use these reactions as a guide to the roles he was being assigned, and to the unspoken parts of the narrative that defined the therapeutic relationship. Initially, he did not speak of these events and reactions, instead choosing to work at maintaining a stance of empathy and interest. These feelings were genuine and were experienced in concert with the anger, defensiveness, and distance that James provoked. Eventually, these enactments, as well as the ways that James unwittingly worked to re-create his life story in the here and now with the therapist, were discussed openly as they occurred.

As this interaction moved along, James began more and more frequently to bring historical and contemporary reports of his life into the therapy, and to lessen his attacks on the process. He slowly became interested in the therapist's opinions about the ideas that had surfaced in the sessions, and also, on occasion, he asked for advice. This behavior gradually moved patient and therapist into an explicit exploration of the interpersonal isolation in which James had grown up, of the ways in which he had explained his parents' seeming disinterest and distance, and of the machine narrative that he had scripted in order to shield himself from loneliness, despair, and isolation.

As these themes became more explicit, James was able to acknowledge his wish for contact with the therapist. This wish was interwoven with themes from the past that conveyed the narrative unit in which James portrayed himself as unlovable and as doomed to "turn to garbage" anything that he hoped for in interpersonal relationships. This piece of the narrative became most explicit and became the focus of much therapeutic work when James announced that he had decided to end therapy to be able to spend more time at work. This decision was announced just after some important gains had been made on unfinished business with his mother through the use of powerful experiential techniques (see Chapter 7 for a more extensive discussion).

James informed the therapist of this decision in a matter-of-fact way and seemed puzzled by the therapist's decided emphasis on extending the discussion of the decision, and by the therapist's evident anger and disappointment. However, as the sessions that followed played out, James became almost gleefully happy and simultaneously and deeply sad. These emotions were explored with a range of techniques that led to the realization that James still had not been able to revise his story to include the therapist as truly liking him and valuing their relationship. James was able to recall instances in his past when he had don foolhardy and dangerous things to provoke his parents into proving that they loved him and were concerned about him. This testing (Weiss, 1994) was repeated in his interaction with the therapist. The therapist's emotional responses and refusal to give up and to "let me go without a fight" strongly contradicted the core pathogenic elements of James's life story.

As time went along, it became clear that the therapeutic relationship had become the source of experiences that James became more and more able to mine and to weave into a new, corrective narrative in which he could portray himself as worthy of love, friendship, and the interest of others. Of course, this narrative also contained tentative characterizations of others as interested, giving, and protective. The construction of this new story also allowed James to revise his view of his own history: No longer did he see himself as having been unaffected by his parents, or as a "mutant" who had never felt any need for intimacy.

There was a great deal of back and forth in the collaborative aspects of the therapeutic interaction. Though James's skepticism and intellectual refutation of psychotherapy diminished greatly, it reappeared periodically throughout the length of the therapy. Over time, both parties came to share the view that the reemergence of James's need to debate signaled a new and painful element of the tale of his life, as well as his reluctance to try to change that plot or to feel the anger, hopelessness, or grief that was part of the story. On a couple of occasions, active cognitive and behavioral interventions were used both to change problematic thinking and patterns of action and to demonstrate concretely the therapist's effectiveness and interest in being of use to James. The gains from these techniques were thus incorporated in tow the creative construction of the subplot in James's narrative that concerned himself and the therapist, countering his pessimism and isolation.

Eventually, James came to describe his interaction with the therapist as a kind of "metaphoric reparenting." He began to try out new ways of relating in the sessions: He told jokes, sparred verbally, and requested experiential and behavioral techniques and assignments to overcome particular problems. James also began to lend the therapist books, to recommend movies and restaurants, and to discuss sports, current events, and a wide range of intellectual topics. He was excited by the therapist's receptivity, enjoyed being able to influence and to teach the therapist, and learned (with the help of some cognitive restructuring and assertiveness training) to confront the therapist when James felt hurt, slighted, or ignored. James described these interactions as the raw data out of which he was constructing a broadened, complex, and favorable image of himself, and he portrayed the therapist as the father of a young adult who encouraged his son's explorations while offering a safe haven and guidance through sometimes rough waters. These events allowed the therapy to move into a final phase that was concerned with the expansion of James's newly constructed narrative to the broader social world.

Insight, Interpretation, and Unconscious Processes

THE ROLE OF INSIGHT AND INTERPRETATION IN TRADITIONAL THERAPIES

Insight and interpretation have been synonymous with psychoanalytic psychotherapy since the earliest days of that method's existence. Once Freud (1900) abandoned his initial reliance on hypnosis and suggestion as ways of helping his patient's toward a cathartic experience, he began to rely on the inferential method, which perhaps defines the classical psychoanalytic method of informing patients about the unconscious meanings of their associations.

Insight was discussed in Chapter 3 as one of several psychotherapeutic change processes. In psychodynamic psychotherapy, it remains the central, and often exclusive, process that is considered responsible for therapeutic gains. Interpretation is the critical therapeutic activity and responsibility of the psychodynamic psychotherapist. Simply defined, a psychoanalytic interpretation is a verbal act in which the therapist tells the patient something about her or his psychological life and experience that the patient does not know. An accurate interpretation leads to insight, which is defined as the patient's being able to know and to acknowledge some previously warded-off and unconscious motive, emotion, moral issue, fantasy, or fear, and the specific interpersonal relationship in which that dynamic originated. "Making the unconscious conscious" is the equation that analytic work attempts to follow before all others.

Insight is both a psychological process and an immediate experience. The term refers to both the mental content that the person first knows, and to the achievement of this new knowledge. In the strict psychoanalytic sense, *insight* refers to conscious acceptance of previously warded-off, and therefore unconscious, aspects of intrapsychic life. The most important mental contents into which the patient may gain insight are wishes, affective states, representations of the self and of others, and the anxieties and prohibitions against becoming aware of these parts of one's psychology. Insight is usually discussed as being accompanied by affective release or catharsis, and by a rearrangement of the intrapsychic structures that govern mental activity. As the person faces what has previously been forbidden to or too frightening for consideration, those issues are redefined as safe, acceptable, and useful, and the realm of psychological possibility expands.

Insight is considered curative because awareness of one's motives, conflicts, and fears allow them to be integrated more fully into the personality, lessens the need for defensive activity, and allows the person to modify or to give up the old anxieties, guilt, shame, and other dysphoria connected with a leftover wish, self-image, or perception of another person. As many writers have pointed out (e.g., Dollard & Miller, 1950; Wachtel, 1977), interpretation and insight provide extensive opportunities for exposure and deconditioning of previously reinforced connections between motivational states, constructions of experience, and anticipated fears. Other analysts have emphasized the new learning experiences that occur in the therapeutic relationships that are catalyzed by interpretation and also on which interpretation depends. In this view, interpretation and insight are part of a larger interpersonal event that leads to psychic restructuring and to the establishment of new and beneficial representations of the self and of others. The analyst who calmly points out a patient's unconscious rivalry with the patient's father and with the analyst becomes a model of acceptance of that emotional state. As the patient learns of those motives, he or she also has the living image of the analyst's comfort and acceptance with which to identify. That interaction is thought by many analysts to lead to positive changes in the patient's conscience and ideal self-image (Strachey, 1934), and to the replacement of pathological object ties with more supportive and healthy internal relationships (Loewald, 1960).

Interpretation requires fluency by the therapist in translating or decoding the patient's conscious reports into meaningful statements about unconscious dynamics. Inference is the key method here, as guided by each therapist's unique version of psychodynamic theory.

The many variants of these theories differ essentially in what they prescribe and proscribe for interpretation: Freudian theory emphasizes repressed sexuality and aggression; Sullivanian theory looks at issues of intimacy, security, and satisfaction; object relations theories frame interpretations around the patient's need for nurturance from others; and self psychological interpretations stress the patient's need for recognition, admiration, and pride. There are many other interpretive systems as well.

Contemporary psychodynamic thinking has questioned seriously the ubiquity and efficacy of insight and interpretation in the creation of therapeutic change. These writers follow in the tradition of such analysts as Ferenczi and Rank (1924) and Alexander and French (1946) who stressed the need for new interpersonal learning (the "corrective emotional experience") in and outside the therapeutic relationship. Their analytic successors, who have most prominently included Winnicott (1971), Kohut (1977), Levenson (1983), Mitchell (1993), Weiss (1994), and Gill (1994), have repeated the view that new experience in the analytic situation is critical in allowing the patient to move beyond old, maladaptive patterns of living. The therapist's immediate ways of interacting with the patient take center stage in these therapies, and the goal of treatment is much more existential than it is exploratory: Patient and therapist endeavor to create a more authentic and real pattern of relating, in the hope that the patient will be empowered to extend his or her newly found authenticity into relationships with others. Interpretation sometimes assists in the creation of this new experience, but often, insight is the consequence of active change on the patient's part. As Mitchell (1993) pointed out, in these versions of psychodynamic therapy, interpretation is considered a complex interpersonal act that impacts upon the patient in many profound ways. The provision of insight is only one of these influences, and it is often not the most important one. Interpretations can be used to help the patient to feel safe, and to feel understood, to challenge pathological behavior, to nurture, to excite, or to comfort. Often, the effect of such interpretations is profound' even if the patient gains no new awareness of his or her wishes, fears, or means of viewing experience.

Among therapists of other orientations, insight and interpretation are found to be most congenial by existential workers (Bugenthal & Kleiner, 1993). This is not surprising since this school of thought has strong theoretical and historical links to psychoanalysis, certainly sharing an emphasis on the expansion of consciousness as a critical change factor. Existentialists depart from classical analysts and, interestingly, converge greatly with more radical contemporary analysts (Gill, 1994; Mitchell, 1993) in what they interpret. These therapists tell the patient of the ways in which he or she deadens and invalidates authentic experience and substitutes culturally derived roles that emphasize comfort at the expense of meaningful living. They speak of existential concerns such as the fear of isolation, meaninglessness, and death, and of the pain of recognizing one's limits and mediocrity.

The use and role of interpretation and insight have been openly denied, if not attacked, by most client-centered and Gestalt therapists. Client-centered therapists avoid interpretation because it is directive and is based on the (untenable to them) premise that the therapist knows more about the patient than the patient herself or himself does. Insight is generally considered much too intellectual a process, which does not assist the patient in expanding awareness and emotionally charged experience (Rice & Greenberg, 1991; Rogers, 1961).

Gestalt therapists also avoid directly telling the patient anything about herself or himself. Applebaum (1981) suggested that the reason is the emphasis on the "how's" of behavior instead of the "why's," as well as the Gestalt preference for work with what the patient is aware of. Gestalt therapy shares with client-centered therapy the aforementioned distrust of the intellectual nature of insight. Both systems of therapy avoid any theoretical inclusion of, or clinical reliance on, notions of a dynamic unconscious, preferring instead to investigate shades of experience and awareness. As a result, interpretation and insight are again rendered relatively useless.

Cognitive-behavioral therapists also eschew the use of these change processes and interventions for theoretical, ideological, and clinical reasons. There is of course no room in these systems for psychodynamic issues, though schema-based cognitive therapies come close to admitting such concepts into their models (Beck, Freeman, & Associates, 1989; Stein & Young, 1992). The action orientation of these therapies; their reliance on instruction, practice, and overt change processes; and the emphatic antipsychoanalytic ideologies of some of the therapies in this group (see, for example, Wolpe, 1958)—all leave little doubt about the lack of importance of insight and interpretation. The use of a psychodynamic formulation or method would be the most heretical act possible for a traditional behavior therapist, since most of the ideas and interventions in this school were formulated in direct opposition to psychoanalysis (Eysenck, 1960; Salter, 1949).

In practice, however, the picture becomes more muddied than these groups of theorists and therapists might have us believe. For example, in viewing recent videotapes of cognitive-behavioral therapy (Goldfried, 1994) and client-centered therapy (Raskin, 1994), my students and I were struck by statements made by these therapists that explained the patient's behavior. Comments were made such as "He's sounding more and more psychodynamic," or "How did he sneak that one in?" Similarly, when reading case reports in the humanistic and behavioral literature that go back as far as Wolpe (1958) or Rogers (1961), one once again sees how central explanation can be to the process of treatment. Often, explanation is silent; that is, it serves as a map for the therapist to consult on the way to suggesting an intervention. But at times, it is overt and violates the rules that were discussed above. Apparently, the need or wish to explain clients to themselves is powerful enough to cause even true believers to cross ideological barriers.

THE VARIED ROLES OF INSIGHT AND INTERPRETATION IN INTEGRATIVE THERAPIES

The extent to which insight and interpretation play a role in the integrative psychotherapies depends largely on the impact of psychoanalytic or existential theories and techniques on each specific therapy. Those therapies that eliminate this influence completely are understandably little concerned with the recovery of unconscious memories, conflicts, and constructions of experience. The many integrative approaches that do include the expansion of consciousness to include previously warded-off psychic contents can be grouped into five fairly distinct perspectives concerning the change value of insight and the technical role of interpretation.

Traditional Uses of Insight in Integrative Psychotherapy

Traditional use in this context refers to the reliance on insight and interpretation in ways that are similar, if not identical, to the process of standard psychodynamic psychotherapies. The therapist listens carefully to the patient's verbal reports, observes the therapeutic interaction, and constructs an inference about some as-yet-unknown conflictual constellation of wishes, fears, self- and object representations, and defenses. This construction is then offered for the patient's consideration. If this presentation is successful, the patient is assisted in integrating these aspects of his or her experience in a personally meaningful way. Greater psychological freedom and a deepened variety of experience is then possible (Mitchell, 1993).

Like sectarian psychoanalysis, the integrative therapists who share this perspective consider insight a central (though certainly not the only) source of therapeutic change. Generally, it is the most frequently relied-on change process, with interpretation sharing this status in terms of frequently used techniques. When other change processes or corrective experiences are deemed necessary, this group of integrationists freely employs active methods drawn from behavior therapy, cognitive therapy, systems approaches, and humanistic therapy. However, these writers (e.g., Curtis, 1993; Frank, 1990, 1993; Gold & Stricker, 1993; Hellcamp, 1993; Rubin, 1993) reserve active methods for situations in which insight is necessary but not sufficient for change. Active interventions are suggested when the patient appears to need to unlearn a symptomatic way of functioning, may benefit from active involvement in a novel, corrective experience, may be helped by the shaping of new adaptive skills, or is so resistant that insight and interpretation have not been helpful. Unlike some of the integrationists who will be discussed below, these therapists do not frequently use active methods to help the patient to become aware of repressed material, or to make that material more easily tolerated consciously. This choice reflects a theoretical bias that construes interpretation as the most direct and powerful way to inform the patient about some warded-off conflict or construction of experience.

Unsurprisingly, this group of integrative therapies displays more resemblance to "pure" psychoanalytic psychotherapy than does any other group of dynamically influenced integrative treatments. Therapies that fit into this perspective actually seem to be fewer in number than those connected with the next three perspectives that we will review. The probable reason is the emphasis on new experience as a change factor that is shared by many integrationists. Also, in part, it may be a historical and professional artifact. Informally, it seems to me that most integrationists started their professional lives as cognitive-behavioral, humanistic, or systems therapists and, over time, came to consider psychodynamic issues theoretically relevant and clinically helpful. The number of psychoanalysts who have moved towards an integrative position seems to be much smaller, hence the less frequent inclusion of traditional insight as a change process in integrative writings.

Insight as a "Cognitive Map" for Change

Some integrative therapies are very little concerned with the patient's gaining a new awareness of, or access to, his or her unconscious life; yet the process of the therapy relies heavily on the therapist's inferences about those issues. As noted above, many Gestalt, cognitive-behavioral, and client-centered therapists seem to use insight in this way. Essentially, these therapies depend on the therapist's insights and use them as a framework for guiding and suggesting active experimentation with new behaviors, cognitions, interpersonal engagements, and affective expressions. Sometimes, these insights are made explicit to the patient and both parties operate from a shared understanding of the unconscious dynamics that will be worked with indirectly.

Deeper change in unconscious motives, conflicts, and representations of experience are assumed to occur gradually without being discussed or focussed on with any great frequency or intensity. The therapy may end with this deeper change having gone unmentioned by both participants; yet these gains are highly desired (at least by the therapist) and are usually thought to be necessary if the active gains and modifications in functioning are to be retained over time.

Cognitive analytic therapy (CAT; Ryle & Low, 1993) is among the most important examples of this mapping use of insight. Technically, CAT relies almost exclusively on work with the patient's overt cognitions and behaviors via the principles and methods of cognitive restructuring and behavior therapy. However, the goals and interventions that are suggested are guided by the therapist's formulation of the patient's unconscious, internal object relations, motivational conflicts, and developmental history. These psychodynamic variables are operationalized in everyday terms, are communicated to the patient in letter form, and are systematically targeted for active intervention.

Westerman's (1993) hermeneutic version of integrative psychotherapy also endorses the view of insight as a topography for change. He argued that knowing how and why we have come to behave as we do is reassuring and stabilizing and corrects of inherited distortions about ourselves and others. However, in themselves, these influences are usually not sufficient to lead to a completely successful therapy. Similarly, change without a map of the patient's unconscious life and history may be superficial or misguided.

While not specifically built around psychoanalytic concepts, the cognitively informed integrative systems advanced by Safran (Reeve et al., 1993; Safran & Segal, 1990) and Guidano (1991) are concerned with the restructuring of deeply embedded, unconscious representations of the self and of others that must be synonymous with issues covered by psychoanalytic theories of object relations. Both of these therapists have used their formulations of the person's unwitting construal of the self and of significant others to guide the selections of cognitive, behavioral, and interpersonal interventions. They have also both been deeply concerned with the use of the therapeutic interaction to create new experiences for the patient, out of which grow both new adaptive, interpersonal skills and important modifications of the unwitting ways in which the patient construes, represents, and retains her or his experiences of the self and others.

This use of insight and interpretation is apparently acceptable to Lazarus (1989), that ardent critic of psychoanalysis. While he has denied that he ever using psychodynamic concepts or methods, his case examples leave no doubt that he has sometimes skillfully framed his interventions with such a perspective, for example, when he has made links between unacknowledged anger and certain behavioral inhibitions and symptoms. This point has been made to me repeatedly by my (admittedly psychodynamically biased) doctoral students, who, on reading a multimodal text by Lazarus (1989), found his disclaimers incomprehensible. These students have kept on pointing out the ways in which Lazarus's sensitivity to latent aspects of the patient's communication served to organize the therapeutic focus and to serve as the springboard for interventions. Some of the more ardent adherents of psychoanalytic theory have even suggested wistfully that they wished their analysts were as perceptive!

Prescriptive Uses of Insight and Interpretation

Without having conducted any rigorous or entirely valid survey, I have made an educated guess that this perspective is the modal one with regard to the place of insight and interpretation in the integrative therapies. Here, enhancing the patient's capacity for self-knowledge and helping him or her to access disowned aspects of experience are valid therapeutic possibilities that take their place among many potential change factors. Some of the integrative therapies that are included in this perspective rely explicitly on the theories of psychotherapeutic change that were reviewed in Chapter 2. These systems include Beutler's prescriptive psychotherapy (Beutler & Hodgson, 1993), Prochaska's transtheoretical psychotherapy (Prochaska, 1995; Prochaska & DiClemente, 1992a, b), and Beitman's (1992) common-factors approach. Prescriptive systems suggest that insight will be more-or-less helpful to each individual, depending on such factors as the person's unique form of pathology, psychological strengths and resources, and readiness for change, as well as the stage of change at which therapy is begun. As a result, some therapies conducted by therapists who adhere to these models use interpretation and rely on insight not at all, while other treatments within the same framework feature moderate or major amounts of such work. Prochaska (1995) pointed out that patients who begin therapy at the stages of precontemplation and contemplation probably require and will benefit more from insight-oriented work than will those people who start therapy already poised for active experimentation with new ways of functioning. Beutler and Hodgson (1993) prescribed insight-oriented work for those patients who repress and deny desires, affects, fantasies, and images of the self and others, while emphasizing that work with unconscious processes may be useless or counterproductive for patients who are depressed, undercontrolled in the face of anger or anxiety, and overly intellectualized and unemotional.

Other integrative systems employ the selective, prescriptive use of insight and interpretation as guided by their unique systems of personality functioning and of the structure and maintenance of psychopathology. For example, in Andrews's (1993) active self model, insight and interpretation are indicated clearly at three stages of the cycle of self-confirmation. Specifically, Andrews advocated the use of interpretation to make the patient aware of unconscious self-conceptions (Stage I), disowned motivations (Stage IIa), and unacknowledged emotions (Stage VIIb). McCullough's (1993) integrative short-term psychotherapy employs interpretation to assist the patient in becoming conscious of pathogenic attributions of causation of behavior and of the ego-syntonic (that is, congruent with some image of the self) nature of certain maladaptive ways of living, and to enhance the patient's sense of competence and mastery by making unconscious experiences and defenses more acceptable, flexible, and adaptive. Allen's (1993) approach aims at the integration into consciousness of previously unacknowledged altruistic motives and positive feelings toward family members in order to reduce and eliminate negatively tinged self-images, self-hating attitudes, and the self-destructive behavior that follows from those intrapsychic states.

These writers share the notion that the change process of insight and the therapeutic method of interpretation are not inevitably linked. That is, even when greater access to previously unconscious issues is the central focus of the therapy, there many be several or many ways to reach that goal. As we noted above, psychoanalysts since

Alexander and French (1946) have observed that insight often follows behavioral change and new experience. Prescriptive integrations have utilized this observation, and they frequently employ active methods other than interpretation to interrupt defenses, reduce resistance, and increase the patient's access to her or his own inner life. Powell (1986) pointed out that exposure-based techniques, such as desensitization, can reduce a patient's anxiety sufficiently so that old defenses can be abandoned and the patient can thus tap into and integrate the unconscious issues that were implicated in the original symptoms. This point was made by McCullough (1993) in describing active restructuring of defenses, and by this writer (Gold, 1993a) in a consideration of the integrative therapy of panic disorders and phobias. Andrews (1993) noted that previously unknown self-images, motives, and emotions can become conscious and lose their disturbing impact when the therapist conveys empathic understanding, prizing, and warmth. Newirth (1995) suggested that the link between intrapsychic change and narrow models of interpretation is far from clear, and that the ongoing interaction of therapist and patient is in itself a more efficacious "interpretation in action."

Similarly, those who integrate individual and systems approaches (Allen, 1993; Kirschner & Kirschner, 1993; Wachtel & Wachtel, 1986) have pointed out that changes in interpersonal relatedness often lead to intrapsychic restructuring and access to previously unconscious feelings, images, and fears. As others in the patient's life behave differently, the ways in which the patient uses his or her own patterns of engagement to ward off self-knowledge are interrupted.

This notion of the multidirectional path to insight unites the writers of this perspective with integrationists who take alternative perspectives that will next be considered.

Insight as a Consequence of New Experience

In this perspective, we find great overlap, if not an amalgam, of the two preceding perspectives. Inferences about the contributions of unconscious functioning serve as a map for interventions, and active techniques are used to enable the patient to integrate and gain access to these issues. Most of the writers who work within this viewpoint share a concern about the roles of exposure and extinction of anxiety as central change processes. These writers, including such contributors as Stampfl and Levis (1967, 1976), Rhodes (1984), Powell (1988), Wolfe (1992a, b); Fensterheim (1993), and Fitzpatrick (1993), agree that unconscious memories, construal, and conflicts must become conscious in an affectively charged way to allow the anxiety-generating meanings of those issues to be extinguished. Defenses, behavioral inhibition, and faulty patterns of relatedness protect the person from exposure to these intrapsychic states. These writers argue that, frequently, interpretation is not effective in producing exposure even if the person cognitively accepts the content of the interpretation. The reason is the power of ongoing action patterns to limit the impact of new information. These ways of living act as an impenetrable suit of armor, which the verbal contribution of the therapist bounces off. Or the therapist's observation is heard without affect or meaning and is assimilated into the web of the patient's ongoing, dysfunctional tale. In fact, very often, the patient's inability to make use of traditional means of interpretation confirms and reinforces conscious and unconscious aspects of the narrative in which the patient portrays himself or herself as hopeless or defective. So, active means are required to produce new intrapsychic configurations that allow exposure to take place.

In these therapies, as in the therapies described in the section on cognitive mapping, interpretation is a precondition of and a map for guiding efforts at change. It serves the therapy by allowing the therapist to construct some behavioral, interpersonal, or cognitive strategy that goes beyond conscious, symptomatic change to underlying areas of experience. Implosive therapy, as discussed by Stampfl and Levis (1976), provides one example. They believe that many patients suffer from repressed memories of traumatic events (abuse, loss, etc.) that produce other symptoms. Implosive techniques involve the combination of the behavioral method of flooding (the prolonged exposure, in imagery, of the patient to the object of her or his fears) with a psychodynamic formulation of the issues that the patient has disavowed or repressed. Phobic patients are exposed not to the actual object of which they are consciously afraid, but to images that approximate the memories, affects, wishes, and fears that are inferred (by the therapist) to be at the root of the symptom. As the process of implosion enables the patient to tolerate what was previously avoided, this material and related memories, images, and affects are made conscious.

Beier (1966), Feather and Rhoades (1972a, b), Fensterheim (1993), Fitzpatrick (1993), and Gold (1990b, 1993a) all offered similar examples of the integrative, psychodynamically oriented use of methods such as systematic desensitization, assertiveness training, and guided imagery to reduce anxiety, and to enhance exposure by preventing the use of previously effective methods of avoidance and escape. As a result, guided by therapist inferences about causal psychodynamic states, the patients became aware of previously warded-off sexual, aggressive, and dependent feelings.

The Cyclical Use of Interpretation and Insight: Toward a Seamless Integration

The cyclical perspective is perhaps the broadest and most inclusive of all five, because it encompasses the views expresses in all of the others just reviewed. Its chief exponent is Wachtel (1991, 1993; Gold & Wachtel, 1993). He, more than any other integrationist, has been concerned with the wording of interpretations, the finer and more subtle aspects of their application, the ways in which the gains suggested by insight-oriented work may be maximized, and the place of insight within a cyclical, multifaceted theory of change.

Wachtel (1977, 1993; Gold & Wachtel, 1993) has suggested that insight can be an independent or dependent variable in psychotherapy: It can bring about change or be brought about by change. Similarly, interpretation can be the agent of change (by making unconscious factors conscious) or can explain changes after they have occurred, thus consolidating a new way of functioning by offering the patient an intellectual framework in which to understand a new experience. Insight can be the therapist's map, used to guide the patient toward an exploration of new behaviors and interpersonal attitudes.

Wachtel (1977) made a uniquely important contribution in his study of the effects that interpretation can have on the patient's experience that go beyond insight. He explained that the wording of an interpretation can offer positive reinforcement of new experiences, such as a willingness to face old anxieties and conflicts, or can be used to prevent the use of a defense or a pattern of avoidance. This latter is accomplished by pointing out those efforts or by discussing them in a way that changes their reinforcement value for the patient. Wachtel pointed out further that interpretations can include hints of new ways of being that may shape new skills and behaviors and can teach people about the behavior of others as well.

A NARRATIVE-BASED APPROACH TO THE INTEGRATION OF INSIGHT AND INTERPRETATION

Human beings seem to have an intrinsic, and perhaps evolutionarily determined, need to understand themselves and the world. Just ask the parents of any bright 3- or 4-year-old how many hundreds of questions, all beginning with why, they answer in the course of a week. The great myths, theologies, and sciences of the past and present have all aimed at explaining the workings of the mind, of nature, and of the spiritual. The art of the interpretation of underlying meanings is part of every society and culture, though Freud and psychoanalysis were perhaps the first to explore this field in a fully systematized way. For example, the Old Testament contains among the first reports of dream interpretation: Joseph, the captive Hebrew slave, rises to the top of Egyptian society because of his facility in finding the meanings of the dreams of the pharaoh. As we saw earlier, the impulse to explain the psychology of the other even seems to extend to those therapists whose ideologies forbid this activity.

It may be that the task of psychotherapy, as Sass (1988) suggested, involves standing behind the individual, to read with him or her the text that is guiding that person's life. If this is the case, we must engage in the search for meanings within that text that the person fears, has learned to avoid or to overlook, or has never had the opportunity to formulate and symbolize.

Storytelling and narrative invariably include an attempt by the author to explain the why's of the behavior of the self and of others. At the beginning of any psychotherapy, the patient has some story about his or her life that has been constructed out of real experiences, fantasies, received opinions, and observations of the self in relation to others. A troubled person is ruled and "lived" by this story without necessarily realizing the impact that this narrative has on his or her behavior and experience. Generally, the story of which the patient is aware at the outset of the therapy is only partially consistent with the story that is perceived by observers of his or her behavior. Often, it is the dim appreciation of the fact that one does not know the whole of one's story that initiates contact with a therapist.

Messer (1992) suggested that this view of psychopathology falls within the "tragic worldview," a perspective on the human condition that posits unknown passions and fears within the person that rule his or her path through life. Unlike the traditional psychoanalytic explanations of the power of the tragic view in explaining and changing behavior (where drives and endogenous wishes are the unknown), the integrative, narrative correlate of the tragic view suggests that the parts of the story that the person tells (by enacting them) but does not know are critical to his or her suffering and to any hope of change.

Most patients are unhappy with their lives and come to us with a sense of passive resignation and a feeling of a lack of authentic and vital inner directedness and autonomy (Shapiro, 1989). Their status in life is quite similar to the characters in Pirandello's play *Six Characters in Search of an Author*, whose aimless and eventually disturbed behavior is explained to the audience as arising out of the absence of a plot and a playwright.

To the degree that any person cannot or will not know the basic stories, or critical parts of those stories, that guide his or her life, that person's experience will overlap with Pirandello's hapless subjects. At the start of therapy, the therapist takes a role quite similar to the audience at this play: He or she observes the plight of the person without a complete story and is eventually drawn into the task of assisting in writing the play. Hopefully, the therapist will have more success in establishing an effective joint authorship than do members of the audience. The characters in this play do not know that their story is of having no story, and without that knowledge, they are doomed to experience themselves as forever remaining without one.

Insight is a powerful change principle in psychotherapy because the act of knowing one's story is in itself a change in the story: The role one assigns to the self in the story is fleshed out historically and experientially, and a sense of active agency and freedom is usually gained. These changes accrue from the person's gradually gained awareness of how and why he or she repeats parts of the story purposely or ironically (Gold & Wachtel, 1993); how and why certain wishes, images, feelings, and thoughts needed to be left unknown; and how a set of scripts—unconscious roles for and characterizations of the self and of others—were constructed, held, and protected from the influence of new learning and experience. As these elements are integrated into the story, new modes of living slowly become available to the person. One can question something that is known and can work at revising assumptions and believes if they are explicit.

Mitchell (1993) suggested that psychopathology is a failure of imagination, in that the patient long ago seized on set ways of viewing and organizing intrapsychic and interpersonal experience. These unimaginative narratives are concrete, rigid, repetitive, and narrow and are put together in ways that admit to no chance of contradiction or change. Some patients (those we may perhaps call narcissistic, borderline, schizoid, or psychotic) may present very unrealistic, elaborate, and fanciful narratives. They simply have another type of deficient imagination for two reasons. First, the degree to which these stories may remove the person from effective connections to herself or himself and to others may be ruinous. Second, when these stories are examined closely, they are revealed to be limited, brittle, and directed to one end: protection of the person from knowing the story she or he fears is real. This unknown story is usually full of danger, damage to the self, unworthiness of love, the unavailability of others, and so on.

With true imagination comes the prospect of new stories that can lead to internal change, behavioral freedom, and vastly novel feedback in one's dealings with others. Imagination requires the capacity to play with and to weave together old and new stories, which contain facts, feelings, hopes, fears, and external events, in their original forms. To do this, one must first be aware of, and be able to act on, the stories one tells oneself, hence the frequent need for therapeutic interventions that undo repressions, denial, and other means of avoiding the unconscious story line.

Insight does more than fill in the gaps in patients' story. It helps them to correct and reduce exaggerations and distortions in their characterization of themselves, their needs and wishes, and the representations or roles that they have thrust on other people. Dangers, weaknesses, strengths, possibilities, and limitations that are assigned to the world, to the self, and to ways of being can be explored, understood, and rewritten. The past, the present, and the future can also be linked and separated more completely and usefully. As patients reconstruct their developmental history, and a new and more complete story of the past emerges (Spence, 1982), new possibilities and story lines become conceivable and may be tested out, with the therapist and with others. This seems to occur because, with a new awareness of how and why we have each written our stories, we also become aware that other scenarios may have been possible or may be even more useful when we considering our past. We also learn that each story is only that: a possible way of constructing meaning from the infinite versions of our life that are possible. Perhaps the "healthy" narrative is one that is taken with a grain of salt by the patient, having been enabled to give up the need to have his or her life story be objectively or historically true (Spence, 1982).

For example, consider the patient who reviews previously unknown aspects of her story, in which she has cast herself as a helpless, guilty, undeserving victim. She may discover points of strength, come to reconsider the role of others in her life in ways that help her rid herself of blame for their actions, and, most important, come to see that other stories might have been possible given different settings and characters. This new knowledge may allow her to look for ways to pursue those new stories, places, and people, thus ending a life of unwitting but tragic repetition.

Interpretation may be used most effectively to provide insight when the patient needs to take in some element of her or his story which she or he does not know but may be ready to hear. That is, therapeutic work has revealed to the therapist some bit of history, motivation, self-image, or other intrapsychic material that will expand the person's awareness of the story without making her or him more uncomfortable that she or he can bear. Narrative-based interpretive work seems to be most effective when a number of conditions are met. The new information is more likely to be heard by the patient when the story of the therapeutic relationship is positive, both consciously and unconsciously, in that old, destructive subplots are not operating. The interpretation will work best if its content does not move the patient too quickly or deeply into a part of the story that she or he still finds too frightening. Similarly ineffective interpretations include those that contradict to too great a degree some self-portrayal or some image of significant people in the patient's life. Finally, interpretation may work best with distorted or warded-off narrative elements that are not associated with skill deficits or lost developmental opportunities. The person may have no good way of changing the story, in spite of increased awareness of it.

When a change in a story line may be impossible because of the increased dysphoria and resistance associated with that narrative piece, other methods are necessary. As we considered above, active interventions demonstrate to the patient that new scripts and roles are possible before, or at the same time as, she or he becomes aware of what she or he has avoided. Successful experimentation is a powerful tool in allowing a person to relax her or his fears and to incorporate new information into the story. It also offers the chance to learn new skills that support and integrate changed ways of construing experience. Here we find the use of insight as a map for change, which was discussed earlier, as well as the location of insight as a consequence of new experience.

An analogy may be drawn to the revision of a script through the work of the writer or the director of a play. Sometimes, during rehearsal, new aspects of a character's motivation, emotions, or sense of self may be discovered by the writer, or by the director, who then confers with the writer about revisions in the script. This process greatly resembles the interpretive work of the therapist, who suggests new ways of storytelling to the patient. At other points, dissatisfied with the way the scene is unfolding, the therapist may encourage the "actor" (patient) to improvise, to ignore the script, to change roles, or to play the scene in an altered physical setting. These new events and behaviors may point out the gaps in the narrative, may unearth unacknowledged subplots, and then lead to revisions. This kind of active intervention to enhances a person's ability to know and to change her or his story.

The participation of the therapist in the construction of a revised or novel narrative cannot be overlooked. We must ever be on guard against the dangers of forcing our stories onto the patient. We may be moved to romanticize his or her life; to cast it in tragic, comedic, or ironic terms that do not quite fit; or to unknowingly live out parts of our own story in the telling of a new version of the patient's tale. Therapists must always remember the editorial function that they serve in this process: Insight should not be coercion, persuasion, or overidentification.

CASE EXAMPLE: JAMES

Insight and interpretation played major roles in therapy with James. As he unfolded, told, and demonstrated the tangled and painful story that had guided and had been shaped by his life, other themes and potential revisions started to make themselves known. Within the tale of the "machine" whose goal was to further his mechanization and total independence were incompletely formed but poignant wishes for contact, love, and approval. James did not acknowledge or seem conscious of this part of his narrative, but his reports of his interactions with his colleagues and employers suggested another story: He deeply wished for some sort of mentoring, nurturance, acknowledgment, and affection from those persons whom he had unconsciously equated with his inaccessible and seemingly uninterested parents.

As a collaborative relationship with the therapist slowly developed (see the previous chapter), James began to bring to his sessions much more material about his past and present life, and particularly about his construal of people's reactions to him at work and at home. Themes and scenarios about the impossibility of finding love and acceptance were gradually interpreted, as were the ways in which he disavowed these wishes and the painful affect tied to them through his overinvolvement in his "machine" ideal. These interpretations met with mild to moderate interest on James's part and seemed to allow the occasional recall of previously forgotten events in his life when he had tried to reach his parents in some meaningful way or had tried to provoke a response in them through his academic successes. These recollections were reported in a relatively flat, unemotional way but pointed to a shift in James's view of himself: At times, he was able to recognize that he had been more pained and in need of familial affection than he had thought at the beginning of therapy.

The intellectualized, "machinelike" way in which James approached traditional interpretive work suggested that a technical shift might appropriately further the integration of these new images and portrayals into the story that James was telling. Therefore, a series of experiential exercises was suggested, in which James was encouraged to use the "empty-chair" technique (Greenberg et al., 1993). However, the purpose of this intervention went beyond the very valuable goal of deepening James's conscious access to his emotions. The point here was to use the emotions that might be made accessible to loosen his intellectual approach to his inner life and to provide dramatic new experiences that might serve as the nuclei for narrative revision. In other words, the hope was that progress in accessing emotional experience would validate the insights and interpretations too powerfully for James to deny them or to weave them into his overcontrolled narrative patterns.

These interventions worked as desired. James found himself confronting deep wells of grief, anger, rejection, and loss as he spoke to the images of his parents. Much "unfinished business" was completed (Beutler & Hodgson, 1993; Greenberg et al., 1993), and the process of mourning was begun (see the clinical example in the following chapter). As important, James came face to face with aspects of his experience and history that could not be pushed away or left out of his representations of himself or of his family. These events led to much self-correction and revision whenever he would get back into his machine mode: Often, he would remind himself of the depths of his need and pain when trying to convince himself (and the therapist) of his essential isolation or of his belief that he had a neurochemical predisposition to be affectless and alone. Of this last, there was no evidence that either party took seriously.

Because of this synthesis of the experiential and the interpretive, previously warded-off narrative themes became better established, conscious elements of James's story and created new, healthy narrative themes that allowed James to utilize much more interpretive work about his past, the present, and his relationship with the therapist. At other points active, behavioral and cognitive interventions were suggested with intentions that were similar to those just mentioned. For example, at a later point in the therapy, James seemed to be slipping back into his patterns of overwork and avoidance of interpersonal involvement. When these behaviors could not be usefully explored dynamically, the intervention of response cost was suggested. An imagery exercise was designed in which James was asked to explain his absences from home to his children. This exercise yielded much guilt, shame, and sadness but also allowed James and the therapist to understand the unconscious meanings of work that James had not be able to consider. As he talked in imagination to his children, he began to become aware of how he had re-created with them his own relationship with his father, as well as the depths to which he wanted his boss to be the father he had never had himself. These insights, in combination with some assertiveness exercises and cognitive self-soothing techniques allowed James to take the risk of confronting his boss about the excessive demands placed on him. This confrontation was highly profitable: James learned how valued he was and how quickly his employer would back off. These techniques eventuated in another revision of James's story, simultaneously accompanied by newly remembered scenes of his having felt ineffective and unimportant when trying to influence his parents. The narrative revisions just mentioned included the establishment of a view of himself as a concerned and loving father who would face his anxieties and difficulties in order to protect his relationship with his children, as well as the creation of a portrayal of himself as potent and worthy of respect and concern from authorities.

The therapeutic relationship was another critical source of insight for James, out of which he made changes in his story. Transference interpretation was used, although sparingly, and seemed very powerful, especially when linked to the therapist's reactions to James. For example, at a point late in the therapy, James found he would have to miss several weeks of sessions because he had been given an overseas assignment by his company. He reported this event matter-of-factly and added that he would understand if the therapist could or would not hold his time open for him on his return. When the therapist replied that he would miss James, was happy that James had achieved such a prestigious and exciting opportunity, and would gladly make the usual times available on James' return, James became highly emotional. Both parties thus became aware of James's unconscious fear that he mattered as little to therapist as he had to his parents, who had blithely accepted his many extended absences from home as a teenager and young adult. The therapist's response and the interpretation of James's fears also served as the starting point for incorporating the novel, affectionate aspects of the relationship into James's construal of his life. This type of interchange occurred periodically throughout the course of treatment. They usually resulted in new glimpses of unconscious themes and in the creation or reinforcement of positively toned narrative elements.

As may be imagined from the description of James's character style, the notions of *truth* and *reality* were very important to him. As James came to know more about his life and to consider the retelling of it, he frequently voiced doubts and anxieties about whether this new story was any more true than the one he had brought to therapy. He even sometimes brought the therapist articles from the popular press, and from psychology journals, that debated the accuracy of recall and retrieved memories. These concerns were explored with an eye how James had used his intellectual skills, and to his need to be certain and to disavow basic existential themes of limits, isolation, and essential helplessness with regard to one's fate. We also looked at his fears that his new story was a product of the therapist's benign interest in him. He learned through interpretation and many self-generated insights that he was afraid of the same kind of coercion in viewing the world with the therapist as he had experienced in growing up, when there had been great pressure not to see things as they really seemed to be.

As a result of this work, James was able to tolerate, accept, and sometimes even enjoy the tentative nature of his new narrative, and to appreciate the possibilities for growth that an open-ended, flexible story provided him.

Experiential Interventions

THE TRADITIONAL THERAPEUTIC USES OF EMOTIONAL EXPERIENCE

Each patient comes to psychotherapy of any sort in a state of pain, confusion, or alienation from the self or from the world. Every system of psychotherapy has a particular vantage point with regard to the patient's subjectivity and emotion. Immediate experience and emotion may be a central clinical and conceptual issue with major technical implications, or it may be relegated to a peripheral place in understanding and intervention.

Emotion and experience are two different phenomena, which are often used interchangeably clinically and theoretically. *Experience* is the broader of the two words and refers to the totality of the patient's subjective or "inner" world. Experience is made up of perceptions, thoughts, attitudes, beliefs, and fantasies, images, bodily sensations, and emotions or affects. However, we frequently encounter a separation of the cognitive and linguistically represented aspects of subjectivity (thoughts, fantasies, beliefs, perceptions) and the more elusive "felt" components of inner life. These aspects of experience, which include feelings, wishful and needful urges, sensations, and images, are usually believed to fall under the heading of affective or emotional experience.

Emotional experience is perhaps the most elusive and ineffable of psychological phenomena. Although there are moods that are stable and long-standing, much of human experience is fleeting, is difficult to put into words and to communicate to others, and is a

product of many other complex psychological structures and processes. The "here and now" of experience and affect is conceptualized
and worked with very differently in the traditional schools of psychotherapy.

The immediate experience of the patient, in all of its nuances,
idiosyncracies, and shades of sensation, meaning, and emotion, is the
shared central concern of the humanistic psychotherapies. Client-centered therapy considers the free and unhindered symbolization of ongoing experience the hallmark of the fully functioning, healthy person
(Raskin & Rogers, 1989; Rogers, 1961). Such a person does not need
to distort or avoid the awareness of any thought, feeling, sensation,
or desire, regardless of its affective valence or its social desirability.
Gestalt therapists suggest that the ability to recognize and contact a
pressing internal need or interpersonal encounter, and to fully attend
to shifts in the interactional field and in the body, is characteristic
of the individual who has reached a state of holistic organization
(Perls, Goodman, & Hefferline, 1951). Existential psychotherapy
shares this concern with helping the person to fully develop her or
his capacity to "be in the world" and to live a free, meaningful life
characterized by the ability to be as self-aware as is possible (Bugenthal & Kleiner, 1993; May & Yalom, 1989).

Humanistic therapies take as their primary data the here-and-now
of the person's ongoing experience. They aim at the expansion of the
patient's awareness of what he or she is experiencing at any given
moment. Rogers (1961) wrote that certain experiences cannot be integrated or accepted by the person because her or his self-image
would be contradicted by the acknowledgment of that personal aspect. As a result, the urge, thought, feeling, or behavior is left unsymbolized; that 75, it remains active in the person's mind but is
unknowable in verbal or cognitive terms. Repeated experiences of this
nature lead to a state of tension and of incongruence. Incongruence
is characterized by alienation from the person's true nature, and by
the restriction of awareness. Only those experiences and aspects of
herself or himself that are consistent with the protected self-image
become conscious. Gestalt therapists also point out that the disturbed
person suffers from a habitual restriction of consciousness and behavior because of socialized anxiety. Direct contact with the phenomenology of the environment and the body is replaced by
mechanistic functioning aimed at repeating learned patterns of interaction that are protective and avoidant. The patient remains unaware
of what he or she feels, thinks, senses, and does. Even the basic bodily functions of breathing, posture, movement, vocal quality and tone,

and muscular tension are impacted and lose their freedom and spontaneity. Existential therapists attend to how neurotic anxiety causes people to distort their experience of themselves and the world, and to enter into a mode of inauthentic and mechanical experience.

These experientially oriented therapies all attempt to promote the search for what patients are doing to their level and state of awareness, and for how they limit their awareness of the moment. These therapies are concerned much less about the etiology or history of a person's problems than are dynamic therapies. Thus, interventions are aimed at immediate demonstrations of blocks, avoidances, restrictions, or failures of symbolization of experience in order to broaden and deepen the patient's consciousness. Client-centered therapy relies on the provision of what Rogers (1957) called the "necessary and sufficient conditions for change": a therapist who is genuine and in a state of self-congruence during the therapy session; the therapist's provision of unconditional positive regard (prizing) to the patient; and empathy for the patient's subjectivity and experience, which allows the therapist to communicate with the patient about those experiences. As the patient learns to be more self-aware, incongruence lessens and self-actualization may occur. This state is marked by a self-image that is realistic and flexible, and that promotes the maximal symbolization of experiences.

Rogers's emphasis on the central position of awareness and the free capacity for symbolization has been adapted and expanded by such therapy theorists as Gendlin (1979) and McGuire (1991), who have created a model and method of treatment called *experiential therapy*. This therapy takes as its focus the moment-to-moment variations and nuances of the widest aspects of bodily and psychological experiencing. Gendlin (1979, 1984) has used a variety of techniques to assist the patient in learning to focus on the here-and-now of experience, and to let go of patterns of avoidance and constriction of what is sensed, felt, and symbolized. Gestalt therapy relies on an affectively charged encounter between patient and therapist. The therapist confronts the patient's habitual patterns of behavior and defense and refuses to engage the patient in these repetitive interactions. At such points, the therapist suggests and designs exercises meant to gradually increase the patient's awareness of his or her bodily distortions, interpersonal habits, and identifications and internalized figures and prohibitions that cause anxiety and limit the patient's scope of awareness. These exercises are meant to be tailored to the immediacy of the clinical situation and maybe as simple as asking a patient to focus on the level of tension in a limb as she or he moves, or to listen carefully to her or his timber and tone as she or he speaks. Technique in Gestalt therapy aims at asking the patient to reflect on the here and now, often simply through such questions as "What are you doing at this moment?" The most well-known class of Gestalt exercises involves enactment of an interaction with an internalized other or with a part of the self. This technique is known as the "empty-chair" or "two-chair" technique and involves a discussion in the here and now with the imagined partner. The goal of all Gestalt techniques is contact with the authentic need, feeling, or perception that is being repressed or disavowed through the restriction of awareness (Rice & Greenberg, 1992).

Existential therapy does not have a well-delineated theory of technique. In general, it is characterized by active questioning by the therapist about the subjectivity of the patient, within a charged and mutually open relationship that is meant to heighten the urgency of the process. Bugenthal and Kleiner (1993) likened the stance of the existential therapist to that of a consultant who assists the patient in mastering the process of inner exploration, which they called "searching." They compared searching to free association, and to other means of turning inward, and they suggested that it brings into immediate focus both previously unacknowledged aspects of experience and the resistances to that expansion of consciousness. Confrontation of resistances to self-exploration is a major task of the therapist, and after many repetitions, it may yield understanding by the patient of the sources of such resistances. This insight may allow the resistances to be abandoned, and a major gain in authentic living is then achieved.

Psychodynamic therapy in its most traditional forms treats the patient's immediate experience as only one of many sources of therapeutic data. Affect, feeling, and sensation, when conscious, are considered derivatives of unconscious conflicts between personally unacceptable motives and internalized values and ideals. This theoretical perspective means that the here and now of ongoing experience is of little clinical value in and of itself. Psychodynamic therapy emphasizes the underlying structures, processes, and motivations that form, populate, and limit the person's ability to be aware of emotions, sensations, and desires.

Conscious emotional experiences are understood to be the felt parts of a complex mental representation that includes a motive, an affective piece, and a cognitive or linguistic label (Freud, 1915; Vaillant, 1993). Emotion serves two general and important psychodynamic functions and provides two related but distinct types of clinical information about the patient. Emotions are a key experience against which defense mechanisms and therapeutic resistances are mobilized. They are also intrapsychic reactions to other emotions, and to fantasies, wishes, and thoughts, that the person cannot accept as being part of the self (Freud, 1900). Both classes of emotion are presumed to be more accessible manifestations of the deeper, more unconscious structures of representation that order and give meaning to the data of psychological life (Basch, 1985).

The emotions and experiences that are found to be unacceptable or unsafe are thus the immediate causes of conflict, and of resistance in the therapeutic setting. This primary class of emotions includes sexual desire and arousal; anger, resentment, and rage; jealousy and envy; tenderness, intimacy, and love; dependency and weakness; autonomy and strength; and spontaneous excitement, vitality, creativity, and joyous pleasure. The particular experiences that are conflictual vary from person to person, depending on their individual developmental history. The secondary and reactive experiences of painful affect that are triggered by other experiences include anxiety, guilt, shame, disgust, embarrassment, and humiliation. These affective sources of resistance are products of the person's internalized familial and social values, conscience and morality, and the aspired-to, idealized, and feared or hated images of the self and others. Any inner state, be it a fantasy, a thought, a wish, a perception, or a feeling, is unconsciously evaluated by the person against these standards, structures, and internalized relationships. This evaluation process leads to anxiety or to dysphoric emotional reactions if the initiating inner state being evaluated comes in conflict with the person's self-image, ethics, or values, or if it threatens some stability of relatedness to an internalized other.

The psychodynamic therapist looks for disturbances, gaps, distortions, and exaggerations of ongoing experiences as signs and signals of resistances and of underlying conflicts. The patient who stops feeling, who feels powerfully and unexpectedly at a certain moment, who behaves in a certain mode while denying the meaning or power of this behavior, and who is confused, pained, or cut off from her or his own inner life demonstrates the operation of defenses and resistances. The ways in which the patient transforms new experiences into repetitions of old events or avoids new learning are critical sources of therapeutic data.

Resistances to the integration of emotional experience, as well as the substitution of past patterns for the immediacy of experience, are most immediately observable in the context of the therapeutic relationship and the transference (Gill, 1982, 1994). When the here and now is studied most carefully, it is in the ongoing interaction between patient and therapist, with an eye toward what is added, left out, left untouched or unnoticed, or changed and distorted. Resistances of any sort are met by interpretation of the painful affect that pulled for the defense, and by exploration of the standards, values, or aspect of the ideal self-image, or of the object relationship that has been threatened. Finally, interpretive work is aimed at insight into the underlying emotional state or desire that was formerly unconscious. In this work, there are several related aims. The first is the modification of the person's processes and structures of self-evaluation in order to make them more benign and realistic. The second is to broaden the range and depth of emotional experiences that can be integrated into the patient's conscious life. The last therapeutic goal is to change the underlying representations of the self and others that shape the ongoing processing of experience.

More traditional Freudian-oriented psychoanalysis encourages historical reconstruction of the early life events and issues that encouraged conflicts around certain experiential variables. Contemporary versions of psychodynamic therapies (Gill, 1994; Luborsky, 1984; Mitchell, 1993; Strupp & Binder, 1984) are more concerned with the how's and what's than the why's; that is, the identity and nature of the unintegrated affects and the present sources of conflict.

As insight into the interpersonal or intrapsychic meaning of affective experiences is achieved, the person's anticipated consequences of affective expression changes, and this change allows access to consciousness of previously unacceptable feelings. Also, as one's perception of emotions changes through interpretation and new experiences, new emotions come to be associated with current relationships and with the self in action (Mitchell, 1988; Wolf, 1988).

Certain contemporary psychoanalysts have come to positions that place work with the woof and warp of conscious experience in a more central place in therapy. Such work generally falls under the heading of *object relations theory* or *self psychology* (Greenberg & Mitchell, 1983). These authors, who include Fromm (1955), Klein (1971), Winnicott (1971), and Kohut (1980), have studied the processes through which the capacity to experience oneself as fully alive, real, and integrated develops emotionally or goes astray. This psychoanalytic work resembles the humanistic and existential schools of therapy in its emphasis on the person's capacity for spontaneous and vivid experience. These psychodynamic advances are based on theoretical propositions that stress the role of ongoing experiences with others in enhancing or interfering with the capacity for experiential openness and with the ability to tolerate and to integrate a wide range of affects. In addition to insight and interpretation, psychoanalytic therapy of this sort relies heavily on corrective experiences within the therapeutic interaction that may repair early developmental failures and may thus help the person to belatedly build up the necessary internal structures for full emotional relatedness.

Behavioral and cognitive therapists do not operate from grand theories of experience and emotion. Affect, feeling, sensation, and related phenomena are approached pragmatically, within an assessment of the role of such variables for each client. Among the most influential theories of emotion in this orientation is the three-factor theory, first advanced by Lang (1979) and elaborated by Rachman (1981, 1984). The three-factor theory suggests that affect, behavior, and cognition exist as three relatively independent psychological systems. The therapist must assess carefully which of the three systems is marked by disturbance and then, optimally, must intervene within that system. Disturbances of the affect system usually include inappropriate or undercontrolled affective states or responses, which are best treated by direct means of modifying affect. In Lang's (1977) and Rachman's (1981, 1984) view, there is no more than a moderate interdependence between affect and cognition, and therefore, emotion is not a consequence of thought. They have also disagreed with the prevailing view in cognitive-behavioral therapy, which suggests that affect and emotions can best be changed through cognitive meanings.

The conceptualization of emotional experience as subsequent to cognitive processing still dominates mainstream cognitive-behavioral writing. Most therapists who utilize a cognitive-behavioral approach rely on principles gleaned from learning theory (Bandura, 1977), personal construct psychology (Kelly, 1963), classical and operant conditioning, rational emotive therapy (Ellis, 1984), and cognitive therapy (Beck, 1976). This general synthesis yields a view that emotions and sensation are biopsychological responses to endogenous and exogenous stimuli and are produced, structured, and influenced by the person's characteristic modes of thinking and perceiving. The content and structure of the belief systems that structure and elicit affect are to some degree genetically determined (Ellis, 1984) and to some degree shaped through observation, modeling, and vicarious learning (Bandura, 1977) and through interpersonal interaction, reinforcement, and contiguity.

Emotion and subjective experience are the foci of cognitive-behavioral therapy when and if such issues are deemed appropriate and clinically relevant by patient and therapist in collaboration. In a cognitive-behavioral assessment of experiential factors, issues of quantity and quality predominate. That is, emotional experience is looked at in terms of being overcontrolled, undercontrolled, or absent, or as being appropriate in amount and kind to the context in which it emerges. Therapeutic interventions are tailored to address the imbalance or the contextual discrepancy of the patient's emotional behavior. The patient whose rage is undercontrolled may be assisted to learn to be moderately angry and assertive. Or the patient who fears the display of tender emotions will be helped to overcome his or her anxieties and to increase in frequency and intensity the desired feelings and their behavioral correlates.

Rarely is cognitive-behavioral work aimed directly at the here and now of immediate emotional experience. Instead, most attention is paid to the antecedents, correlates, and consequences of emotions. The modification of links between cognitive, behavioral, and situational factors and emotions is the usual goal. For example, in Beck's (1976) cognitive therapy of anxiety or depression, the affective, sensory, and biological symptoms and phenomena are approached via modification of the structuring beliefs and the behaviors that maintain or ameliorate these experiential variables.

Certain behavioral and cognitive techniques and goals are aimed at increasing a patient's access to, and awareness of, immediate experience. In very dramatic ways, self-monitoring and the recording of dysfunctional or irrational beliefs enhance patients' sense of the here and now and their role in their own pathology. As the patients learn to identify, question, test, and revise their pathogenic cognitions, the link between thought, affect, and behavior is made real in an exceptionally vivid way. Patients also experience themselves in an enormously different way. The formerly helpless, depressed, or anxious person becomes empowered and self-efficacious (Bandura, 1977). As one's construal of oneself changes in positive ways such as these, other cognitive, behavioral, and affective changes may follow as well.

In very powerful and immediate ways, behavioral exercises such as assertiveness training, behavior rehearsal, and imagery-based and *in vivo* exposure techniques (e.g., desensitization and flooding) focus patients on their subjective experiences of safety and anxiety, and on affects such as shame, embarrassment, anger, and guilt. Successful utilization of these techniques also helps to patient to experience such affects as transient, tolerable, and changeable.

The here and now of the patient's experience of the therapist is not a central concern of these therapies, but it does become a focus at times, particularly when an impasse or stalemate has been reached. At those times, many cognitive and behavioral writers recommend a careful review of the interaction in order to promote further therapeutic movement.

INTEGRATIVE THEORIES OF EMOTIONAL EXPERIENCE

Two main trends characterize the work of integrative theories of emotional experience. The first trend involves the integration of work from general emotion theory with various approaches to psychopathology and psychotherapy. The second trend in integration is more specific efforts to integrate ideas and methods from different schools of therapy without resort to the more general field of emotion research.

Integrative approaches to emotion that aim to synthesize clinical and empirical findings must consider, and perhaps bridge, the dichotomy between the *biosocial* and the *constructivistic* perspectives on emotion (Izard, 1991). While there currently exist many competing theories of emotions, these theories share certain characteristic that allow them to be placed within one of these superordinate categories. Biosocial theories of emotion (Izard, 1991; Pascual-Leone, 1991) suggest that emotional experience is in part genetically determined and that each individual's biological heritage determines certain qualitative factors of emotional experience, especially the intensity of any particular feeling and the thresholds of affects. Biosocial theories give affect and emotion a central motivating and organizing role in general personality functioning, to which thinking and perception add content and form. Emotions are believed to have many possible antecedents, including conscious cognitive appraisals, subcortical psychological activity that occurs out of awareness, and neurochemical events and processes.

Constructivist theories disregard genetic and biological predispositions and emphasize the ideational and cognitive construction of emotional experiences. Such constructions occur in, and are built of, the interpersonal field and the social environment. More traditional constructivist theories assign emotion the position of a transient dependent variable that is determined solely by cognitive appraisal or other ideationally based variables. Thus, emotions are believed to have little, or only secondary, determining power over behavior or cognitive activity (Izard, 1991).

Integrative theories of emotional experience have been offered that attempt to synthesize the ideas offered in the biosocial and the constructivist theories of emotion. These theories share an evolutionary and adaptive perspective that is drawn from the biosocial perspective, as emotional experience is believed (Guidano, 1987, 1991; Safran & Greenberg, 1991) to derive from humanity's biological heritage and survival needs. At the same time, affective experience is believed to be a form of knowledge about the world that provides rapid and immediately processed information about the environment and the interpersonal field. Such knowledge is in part a reflection of inborn, evolutionarily determined capacities and processes, but in large part, emotional knowing is composed of stored memories, perceptions, and schemas against which new perceptual and visceral data are compared and organized.

Guidano (1987, 1991) has suggested that two types of knowledge grow out of the interaction of evolutionary biological and survival needs with social experience and the human organism's capacity for symbolization and the construction of experience. He referred to emotional experience as the conscious, felt component of *tacit knowledge* processes. Affective or tacit knowledge is experience and action that are produced by the evolutionarily most primitive, ancient systems of information processing, and they are the most spontaneously and in-the-moment kind of "knowing response" (Guidano, 1991, p. 53). The survival value of emotion is a critical point of consensus among integrative therapists (Daldrup, Engle, Holiman, & Beutler, 1991; Greenberg & Safran, 1984). Emotional responding and knowing occur out of awareness and before the conscious direction of attention and concentration can occur. In fact, the information processing that guides and produces emotional experience may be totally automatic and free of the influence of conscious deliberation (Greenberg & Rhodes, 1991).

Tacit, emotional knowledge is necessary to ensure survival. It does so in a motivational and purposeful way by influencing the person's selection of behaviors in a reciprocal relationship with more sophisticated knowing systems of explicit knowledge. The person's survival and adaptive skills are enhanced by affective experience and tacit knowing in several critical ways. Emotions provide the person with information about the consequences of an intended action or behavior. This information is obtained intrapsychically as the person remembers similar intentions and acts. These emotionally charged memories, imagery, ideas, and feelings may serve an inhibitory function if the affects are fearful or in some other way negative. Should neutral or positive emotions accompany one's appraisal of potential behaviors, that intention is likely to be expressed openly. Emotions also assist in making adaptive choices because of their immediacy and salience (Safran & Greenberg, 1991), which tend to focus attention on a limited number of cognitive and behavioral choices at any given moment. The impact of an emotionally toned experience is more powerful and more difficult to ignore than that of more impersonal ideas and opinions, moving the person to act rather than to equivocate or delay where to do so may be dangerous or inopportune.

Emotions offer the self and other persons immediate information about an individual's intentions and current psychological state. Often, the meaning of an event or experience cannot be symbolized or represented completely, if at all, in linguistic or cognitive terms. In introspection, the person will know what she or he is ready to do, or how something has affected her or him, on the basis of a spontaneous emotional response, which gives rise to cognitive meanings only later. The motoric behaviors, vocal tones, and facial expressions that are associated with emotions provide others with critically important information about the person's readiness to respond in specific ways at any given moment. These emotion signs trigger emotional, cognitive, and behavioral responses in these others. Accurate and successful reading of this affective communication assists in adaptive interpersonal decision making, often in a more rapid and influential way than does a purely verbal informational exchange (Safran & Greenberg, 1991; Safran & Segal, 1990).

Integrative theories suggest that the separation of cognition and emotion is artificial and arbitrary (Guidano, 1987; Safran & Greenberg, 1991; Safran & Segal, 1990). Emotion and cognition are considered complementary systems of processing information and of representing and storing experiences. Both systems serve the person in creating meaning of the massive array of sensory, perceptual, and interpersonal data with which the organism is faced. Emotional meaning is highly immediate, personal, and often vague and is concerned with the here-and-now state of the person or the interpersonal situation of the moment. Cognitive meanings are more specific, distant, and abstract and are connected with larger issues and concerns. As many authors have pointed out, cognition fills out temporally, geographically, and biographically the immediate urges and arousal of the affect state. The question of "hot and cold" cognition (Zajonc, 1980) or the need to assign precedence to cognition or to affect as being the antecedent of the other is made obsolete in these writings as well. Most integrative theories suggest that both "top-to-bottom" (cognition leading to emotion) and "bottom-to-top" (emotion eliciting cognition) processing are common, and that, in fact, both processes probably occur simultaneously and are reciprocally influential (Greenberg et al., 1993; Safran & Greenberg, 1991).

Emotional experience is organized into emotional schemas or working models that are complex representational structures (Bowlby, 1980; Guidano, 1987; Safran & Greenberg, 1991; Safran & Segal, 1990). Over the life span, such emotional models are constructed of the raw material of each individual's subjective impressions of his or her interactions with others. The individual develops generic classes, categories, or prototypical ways of representing and remembering other persons, events, and situations. Each memorized model is stored with a specific emotion or set of associated emotions, which are experienced and felt whenever an experience is judged to be similar to a stored emotional schema and thus to bring that schema into an organizing position in awareness. While many central emotional schemas are established early in life within the context of the most salient attachment relationships (Bowlby, 1980; Guidano, 1987), there is also reworking, modification, and revision of earlier emotional schemas as new experience accrues.

The second major trend within integrative psychotherapy is an extension and synthesis of ideas drawn from humanistic-experiential therapy with other therapeutic systems and methods. Experientially based integrative theories are more concerned with the broader concept of experiencing, and with the capacity of the individual to reach the deeper, nonverbal levels of psychological life in a way that promotes growth, adaptation, and an internal sense of completeness. These studies reflect the influence and integration of client-centered and existential therapy with Gestalt therapy (Fodor, 1993; Greenberg, 1992; O'Hara, 1984; Rice, 1984) and with existential therapy, systems approaches, dynamic therapy, and cognitive-behavioral therapy (Bohart, 1990, 1993; Goldfried, 1995). Experience and experiencing are defined by the processes that they contain. As by the integrative emotion theorists discussed above, experience is regarded within adaptive terms as a product of knowing about the self and the place of that self within an environmental context. Experience in the moment arises from the nonverbal processes of apprehending, sensing, and feeling, and it informs the individual about her or his place in the world in a preverbal way. The component processes of experience include bodily sensations and urges; nonverbally sensed anticipations of events, needs, and input by others; images; perceptions of the contextual and environmental field; emotions; and thoughts. The person rarely becomes aware of these constituent processes because of the holistic nature of experiencing when it is unimpeded (Bohart, 1993). Cognitive andverbal labeling of this knowledge, or felt meanings (Bohart, 1990), is the final step in the experiential process that allows these states to be reviewed, remembered, and discussed with the self and with others.

Emotions are understood to be a subcategory of experience and are simply one type of feeling or experiential state that informs the person and others around her or him of the meaning of an event, telling "how" and "how deeply" the person is being affected (Bohart, 1993). Emotions become part of experience when the meaning of something that the person has felt or sensed is personal, significant, and important to that individual. Experientially informed integrative theorists suggest that optimal psychological functioning is marked by a "process orientation" (Bohart, 1990) that allows the person to fully apprehend and sense all aspects of the ongoing flow of experience. As the bodily, ideational, affective, and interactional data of experience register on and are noted and scanned by the person, she or he constructs personal "felt meanings" of these inputs. The well-functioning person is open to an ongoing review of her or his meaning construction and does not get trapped in a absolute, concrete, or rigid relationship with such construals. Such a person lives in a flexible, open, and constantly evolving relationship with her or his ideas, feelings, and behavior and is able to adapt most effectively to new contextual challenges and opportunities. As novel interactions with the environment take place, the person is able to look within and without simultaneously, can listen to the bodily and nonverbal meanings of the event, and is eventually able to synthesize the felt meanings with verbal or symbolic processes. This process involves an internal dialogue between two levels of the person: the level of holistic, felt sensation and apprehension, which knows things immediately but without words, and the level of conscious symbol formation and linguistically based constructions. As a result, when the person finds that her or his ways of interpreting experience have led to problems, she or he can step back, can reconsider and reprogram, and is then able to return to the here-and-now flow of experience (Bohart, 1990, 1993).

Other integrative approaches, in psychodynamic or cognitive theories are the central components, tend to give little emphasis to the place or role of emotional experience. Most of these approaches rely on traditional ways of conceptualizing emotion that relegate it to a position secondary to dynamic, motivational, cognitive, or inter-actional variables. Additionally, most of these systems do not con-sider the here-and-now of the patient's experience a central issue; rather, they see the flow of consciousness as a derivative of other factors. A few notable exceptions should be mentioned briefly.

Psychodynamic theories that integrate interpersonal (Strupp & Binder, 1984) and or cognitive principles view affect as adaptive in-formation about the environment and or as actions or action tenden-cies (Schafer, 1976) in an interpersonal context. Affects are shaped, influenced, and regulated by beliefs, perceptions, and anticipation of their consequences, and such variables may make affect inaccessible (unconscious) or pathogenic (Weiss & Sampson, 1986). Wachtel's (1977, 1993; Gold & Wachtel, 1993) theory of cyclical psychody-namics suggests that emotions may be conscious or unconscious de-terminants of other psychological processes and are also sometimes the consequences of interactional events and patterns of consolidating relationships. In a like vein, Lazarus (1992) included affect and sen-sation as two components of the BASIC ID profile in multimodal ther-apy and suggested that these phenomena may be found at the beginning, middle, or end of a firing order or behavioral chain. Gold-fried (1994, 1995) has expanded his view of the central change proc-esses in behavior therapy to include affective arousal. He noted that research has indicated that pathogenic cognitions and behaviors are more likely to change when the patient is emotionally stimulated. As a result, he has incorporated certain gestalt exercises into his tech-nical repertoire.

INTEGRATIVE INTERVENTIONS

The Role of Emotion and Experience in Integrative Psychotherapies

Emotional health is marked by the capacity to feel emotions freely, without excess or inhibition. A healthy emotional life is also characterized by a quality of emotional responsiveness wherein the person, as well as significant others in his or her life, appraises his or her emotional experiences to be consistent with, and appropriate to, the immediate circumstances in which those emotions are mani-fested. The overcontrolled or affectively out-of-control person, or the person who is angry, fearful, guilty, elated, or sad at unexpected times and in unexpected places, may be demonstrating a pathology of emotional schemas. These aberrant emotions are reflective of and are caused by the activation of emotional schemas of which the person may or may not be aware. Conscious or not, these schemas cause the person to react to the immediate situation in a subjectively determined, seemingly disturbed or emotionally inappropriate manner that may be incomprehensible to that individual or to the observer. When existing emotional models are skewed, limited, and resistant to new experience, the person is biased toward a few predominantly negative affects such as fear, anxiety, or anger.

Experientially oriented integrative work suggests that psychopathology is a result of the loss of a process orientation to experience, or of blocks in the person's ability to engage freshly in experiences in an ongoing way. Defensive activities, the inability to step back and reconsider felt meanings and ways of construing experience, and damage to relations with the self and others are the results of experiential blocking. The person is unable to identify or apprehend new experiences and becomes caught in maladaptive and stereotyped patterns of thinking, feeling, and behaving.

Greenberg (Greenberg et al., 1993; Greenberg & Safran 1984) has suggested that pathogenic emotional processing may manifest itself clinically in any or all of three realms of experience. The person may be unable to become aware of or to integrate and to act on potentially useful and adaptive emotions; may demonstrate automatic, excessive, and repetitive dysfunctional patterns of emotional response; and may experience certain state-dependent reactions that are otherwise inaccessible to intervention (such as being self-critical when depressed). Another important area of emotional dysfunction identified by integrative therapists is "unfinished business with others" (Daldrup et al., 1991; Engle, Beutler, & Daldrup, 1991). This dysfunction refers to a chronically inhibited or blocked emotion that causes an ongoing state of tension and conflict, and that interferes with the person's abilities to behave adaptively.

Complex interactional patterns of failure and avoidance may develop that limit the person's opportunities for new experience. The person's behavioral choices and ability to problem-solve are limited severely by the narrow and repetitive emotional information available, and by the equally small number of salient motivations embodied in these affects. This limited array of behaviors and attitudes may elicit responses from others that are rejecting or hurtful and then may reinforce and confirm existing negative emotional models. Such a process may result in the person's being trapped in a vicious circle of ongoing negative emotional experiences (Gold & Wachtel, 1993; Safran & Segal, 1990; Wachtel, 1977, 1993).

Experiential and emotional change are at the heart of a small but significant group of integrative psychotherapies, which are derived from and based on some of these theoretical positions. These therapies rely on the selective use of techniques and procedures drawn from client-centered, Gestalt, cognitive-behavioral, and dynamic therapy to reach their goals, which include changes in conscious awareness of the narrow category of emotions and the more broad and inclusive category of experience. Different integrationists have identified slightly different taxonomies and categorizations of experiential and emotional change. Greenberg and Safran (1984) suggested that three types of emotional change are central to psychotherapeutic progress: (1) enhancing the patient's ability to identify, tolerate, and use adaptively emotions previously thought and felt to be unacceptable, bad, or dangerous; (2) decreasing the frequency and habitual nature of certain dysfunctional emotional reactions; and (3) modifying cognitive processes and structures that are conscious only during certain affective or mood states.

Greenberg and Rhodes (1991) offered an alternative expansion of this view; they suggested that three crucial components of affective functioning exist in psychotherapy. The first mode, the *historical-interpersonal* modes refers to how the patient's emotional responses to the therapist are colored and determined by the patient's past relationships and by internalized rules, images, and emotional schemas derived from those experiences. The second type of emotional processing implicated in therapy is the *phenomenological mode*, which describes how emotions feel and affect the patient, with particular scrutiny of the patient's ability to focus on specific emotions and to tolerate and use them adaptively. The final type of processing mentioned by these authors is *motivational affective processing*, which refers to the implications for action and the perceived consequences interpersonally that are attributed to emotions by the patient. Greenberg and Rhodes concluded that the goals of an affectively oriented integrative therapy must include the exploration and alteration of the patient's maladaptive expectations about the intrapsychic and interpersonal consequences of emotions, as well as assistance in ridding the patient of the cognitive, dynamic, and attitudinal blocks that cause the patient to avoid, repress, deny, or distort emotional experience.

Safran and Greenberg (1991) offered the most exhaustive review and integration of various dynamic, experiential, cognitive-behavioral, and empirical studies of the role of emotional change in psychotherapy. Their list includes these seven ameliorative affective change processes: emotional restructuring, catharsis, experiential symbolization, facilitating cognitive reorganization, motivating adaptive behavior, corrective emotional experience, and affect attunement. *Emotional restructuring* is the process of contacting and changing the patient's basic ways of responding to and processing information in order to eliminate maladaptive affects, and to promote the development of new emotions. *Catharsis* is a therapeutic principle relied on by many therapies, self-help groups, and other social and cultural experiences and institutions; it refers to the act or process of consciously experiencing and integrating previously feared, avoided, or warded-off emotions. *Experiential symbolization* is a method of personal discovery in which the patient is assisted in translating and deconstructing an immediate problematic emotional reaction into its underlying attitudinal, motivational, schematic, and historical roots and organizing structures. When an affectively heightened interaction between patient and therapist leads to disequilibrium in the patient's ways of thinking, perceiving, and constructing experience, the process of *emotional facilitation of cognitive reorganization* may be inferred.

New capacities for recognizing and accepting previously avoided emotions also cause a shift in the person's interactions with the environment. Because emotions are intrinsically motivating, a more emotionally expanded individual has at her or his disposal a greater motivational array of choices (motivating adaptive behavior.) *Corrective emotional experience* is a concept derived originally from the psychodynamic studies of Alexander and French (1946), and it figures heavily in many integrative therapies (e.g., Allen, 1993; Gold, 1993a, b; Ryle & Low, 1993; Safran & Segal, 1990; Wachtel, 1977). It is defined by an interaction between patient and therapist that breaks, disconfirms, or in some other ways fails to reproduce the patient's characteristic interpersonal patterns and ways of engaging another person. As a result, the patient's typical ways of thinking, feeling, and perceiving are highlighted and interrupted, and new experiential and emotional data may impact on the patient in a novel and creative way. Finally, *affect attunement* is the ability of the therapist to experience and symbolize for the patient, and to communicate to the patient the patient's as yet unknowable and unacknowledged affective states.

Beutler and his colleagues (Beutler & Hodgson, 1993; Daldrup et al., 1991; Engle et al., 1991) have suggested that enhancing the capacity for emotional expressiveness is a central issue in many therapies, particularly when the patient is overcontrolled affectively or is experiencing anxiety, tension, and symptomatic distress because of chronically repressed, inhibited, or denied emotions. These authors have argued that such inhibited affective states are the expression of "unfinished business" with a significant other with whom an ongoing relationship has ended or changed.

Bohart (1990, 1993) has identified the capacities to freely experience one's felt meanings, to evaluate one's construal of experience in a flexible and self-corrective way, and to learn from experience in a creative and open-ended way as principles that are implicated in and are relied on by all forms of therapy. He suggested building an integrated psychotherapy on the framework of experiential freedom as the predominant goal. Bohart (1992) pointed out that experiential learning takes place at both conscious and nonconscious levels and involves a transformations of intellectual and cognitive awareness into a bodily experienced, viscerally felt, and concrete form of knowledge. He argued that psychotherapeutic work that does not address this level of experience is artificial and overly abstract and intellectualized.

Finally, Rice (1984; Rice & Greenberg, 1991) has stated that a successful integrative psychotherapy built on a client-centered foundation is aimed at helping the patient in the reprocessing of cognitive and affective experience.

Technical Approaches in the Here and Now

Given the positions espoused by the writers mentioned above, how do they (and others like them) actually work toward the therapeutic goal of emotional and experiential change? As a first principle of technique, there is substantial agreement among many integrationists that changes in awareness and in experiential processing are best obtained within the context of an emotionally charged, safe, and empathic therapeutic relationship. This relationship meets the three criteria for therapeutic changes outlined by Rogers (1957, 1959) as the therapist responds to the patient in a congruent way, with empathy and with unconditional positive regard. As Guidano (1991) wrote, emotional involvement by therapist and patient in the relationship in the process of therapy is crucial for change. As the discussion of explicit factors in a patient's life cause disequilibrium and a novel opportunity to change experiential meanings and to incorporate new information, involvement on an emotional level ensures that this information is highlighted and is therefore less able to be ignored or distorted.

However, integrative approaches also argue vigorously for an inclusion of more active and evocative techniques that arouse warded-off emotions and experiential states, that point out to the patient and help him or her to overcome blocks in experience, and that foster and promote new learning. The active techniques in these efforts have been Gestalt exercises, guided imagery, behavioral exercises aimed at exposure and social skills training, dynamic interpretation, interpersonal disconfirmation, and many others. In some cases, the specific technique is used directly to bring a new feeling or meaning into consciousness (for example, through a focusing exercise or a Gestalt two-chair dialogue); in other instances, the technique has been adapted to bring into awareness a block to experiencing or some other maladaptive response that can then be unlearned or overcome through some other interventive strategy.

Several important integrations of client-centered and Gestalt therapies have been developed in recent years, often with the inclusion of concepts and techniques from cognitive-behavioral and dynamic therapies (Greenberg & Rhodes, 1991; Greenberg et al., 1993; O'Hara, 1984; Rice, 1984; Rice & Greenberg, 1991). In these integrative models, the therapist works to establish the traditional relationship of client-centered therapy as described above. This relationship in itself is often found to allow for experimentation with emotional expression and disconfirms for the patient expectations of punishment, rejection, humiliation, or other negative consequences for an open emotional display. However, this stance is often insufficient to mobilize feelings and the object representations and cognitive structures that are implicated in blockages and defense.

Rice (1984; Rice & Greenberg, 1991) has added to the client-centered framework an active approach based on the identification by the therapist of certain emotional markers in the patient that signal a need for novel interventions. These markers indicate that patients are at a point of readiness to experience and to reprocess some area of their inner life that has been unsymbolized up to that point. This reprocessing goes hand in hand with the reexamination of older experiences that illuminate and shape the newly symbolized experience. The process markers include mention by the patient of a sense of vulnerability, damage, or difference from other persons (Rice & Greenberg, 1991). Such markers are met with a message that has been described as *empathic prizing* which affirms the humanity and worth of the patient and does not attempt to explore or change the experience in any way. If successful, this intervention leads to a full experience of the vulnerability without avoidance and distortion, but with an incorporation of the therapist's regard, and with a diminution of the anxiety and incongruence associated with the perception of the self as vulnerable. This reprocessing then contributes to an expansion of the self and of awareness and allows the patient to reconsider and test the thoughts, feelings, and experiences associated with the vulnerable image of the self.

A second process marker is the revelation by the patient of some problematic reaction about which the patient feels confusion, discomfort, or shame. Such experiences are the start of a process of experiential searching (Rice & Greenberg, 1991) that gradually enables patients to enrich their conscious experience and to spontaneously come in contact with the affective and cognitive meanings and schemas that guide experience, as well as with the memories and conflicts that gave rise to those structures. The therapist assists in the experiential search in a number of ways. She or he first acts to keep the patient focused on the reaction that is felt to be problematic, rather than on secondary or consequent feelings and thoughts. The therapist then encourages the patient to re-create and reenter the scene of the reaction in as real and as vivid a way as possible, and to report on all sensory and perceptual experiences at that time. This re-creation allows the patient to recapture memories of a nonverbal nature that come closer to the basic emotions and emotional schemas than do conceptual and verbal data. Following these steps, the patient is questioned about the most salient aspect of the occurrence and learns to identify the personal meanings and appraisal were operating but not originally in awareness. Finally, the patient begins to explore the more general characterological and historical significance of the single problematic reaction.

Greenberg (1992; Greenberg et al., 1993) has broadened his integrative therapy into a synthesis of client-centered, Gestalt, and cognitive therapies, which he calls process-experiential therapy. He has taken as his starting point the establishment of the client-centered relationship conditions and has suggested that this relationship is critical in providing a safe haven in which patients can explore their fears about themselves and about their emotional life.

Added to this foundation is the extensive use of active interventions, including especially Gestalt exercises such as the two-chair technique, in which a dialogue is established between the patient and another figure from the patient's past or present life. These exercises, as well as other imagery-based, active techniques, are used to make vividly evident the negative thoughts, feelings, object representations, fantasies, and sensations in a conscious, here-and-now experiential way. As these experiences are played out, other aspects of their components begin to come to consciousness and can be explored. The therapist works in a directive, guided, and suggestive manner, telling the person which exercises to try and when to switch roles or voices, a procedure most useful when blocks or resistances occur. At these moments, the patient is asked to play out both sides of an internal dispute or conflict. As this exploration continues, the therapist continues to respond to the patient in an empathic and unconditionally positive way and tries to offer affirmation and prizing at times when new and more positive states of self-organization and experience are emerging and are being made conscious. The patient's pathogenic modes of emotional and cognitive processing, as well as his or her dysfunctional identifications, self-images, and object representations, are offered correction not through discussion or intellectual review, but through the provision of new and immediate alternative experiences. These new experiences are processed at deep levels of knowing because of their affective charge, and over time they may coalesce into more adaptive emotional schemas and representations.

Another integrative method that leans on Gestalt techniques to intervene in affective problems is focused expressive psychotherapy (Daldrup et al., 1991; Engle et al., 1991). As mentioned above, this therapy is geared toward ending "unfinished business" with a significant other that is causing the chronic repression or inhibition of certain emotion states. The person is unable to identify or apprehend new experiences and becomes caught in repetitive patterns of thinking, feeling, and behaving. The first task of this therapy is the identification of a marker of unfinished business. This marker is manifested in four ways, via (1) an emotion manifested in the present in a lively way; (2) the establishment of a relationship between the emotion and a significant other; (3) the ongoing feeling of blockage, inhibition, or constriction of the emotion; and (4) the awareness of the current problematic nature of this interrupted feeling.

Once the marker is located, the therapy proceeds through five steps. The first step involves establishing mutual agreement on a therapeutic focus and task, while the second step is working to obtain a clear commitment from the patient with regard to entering into and sustaining an imaginal or experimental dialogue or interaction with the significant other. The third part of the therapy is made up of actual engagement of the patient with the imagined significant other in trying out new expressions of the blocked emotions. As this task progresses, usually through Gestalt dialogues, older experiences and images of relationships may emerge. As appropriate, the patient may be encouraged to try out new emotional expressions with these persons as well. This affective experimentation is done on the assumption that these spontaneously recalled relationships represent new access to emotional schemas and processing that were implicated in the block in the person's present life. The fourth and fifth steps in the process involve periodic assessment of the therapy and the development and review of homework assignments and of plans for the future.

Bohart (1990, 1992, 1993) has based his approach to integration on the premise that all psychotherapies aim at and produce changes in the processing of experience. He has suggested that people turn away from experience because of some of its more painful aspects. If pain, in the form of frustration, hopelessness, helplessness, or fear, is too great and too chronic, relatively permanent blocks in awareness are established. These blocks are overcome in Bohart's therapy through identification with the therapist's openness and congruence, and through the healing effects of empathy and positive regard. There are also four technical steps in the therapy that encourage and aid the person in expanding awareness. The first of these is the learning of *experiential articulation*, which refers to providing and attaching words and labels to feelings, sensations, and affects. *Direct experiential learning* is another step, wherein new schemas are learned, and old ones are abandoned or modified as new experiences are provided. *Experiential evocation* refers to techniques that enable patient and therapist to heighten the alive, felt part of any experience, while *habit* refers to the need for massed practice or many trials of learning to change experiential processing. Each step in Bohart's experiential therapy can be accomplished through many intervention possibilities, including dynamic interpretation, experiential focusing, gestalt exercise, cognitive-behavioral procedures, and interpersonal or systemic input (Bohart, 1990). What is crucial is the tailoring of any technique to the experiential block, need, and task at hand.

Safran's (Reeve et al., 1993; Safran & Segal, 1990) approach to experiential change is based on an assessment of the patient's participation in the therapeutic relationship, and on a combination of empathic communication and interpersonal disengagement, which render ineffective the patient's characteristic ways of relating to others and to herself or himself. As the patient's patterns of engaging others are disrupted and understood, the vicious circles of behavior, thought, affect, and schema are undone, leaving the person more open to fresh construal and to creative experience. Safran's therapy depends heavily on the technique of unhooking, which involves a recognition by the therapist of the interpersonal pattern, and underlying schema, with which the patient is attempting to engage the therapist. As the therapist feels pulled into the patient's habitual interaction pattern, the therapist begins to metacommunicate, or to talk about her or his current experience or relatedness vis-à-vis the patient. Metacommunications convey to the patient information about his or her effect on the therapist and the therapist's observations of the patient's nonverbal behaviors and covert communications. As this process unfolds, the patient learns about his or her habitual patterns of interaction, and the therapist is able to disengage, or unhook. In doing so, she or he disconfirms the client's expectations, causing disequilibrium in the patterns of information processing and emotional responding that the patient has brought to the relationship. As a new and potentially healthy experience is constructed between therapist and patient, the patient is more able to turn toward intrapsychic exploration, which is met by empathic understanding and positive regard.

In this therapy, emotional experience, cognitive processing, and interpersonal engagement are considered equally important and inseparable aspects of experience. Therapeutic attention moves from one to the other as the clinical situation dictates, but emotionally charged experiential change is critical for changes in other aspects of experience and is also unlikely in the absence of cognitive modification or without changes in interpersonal behavior. This therapy's emphasis on the circularity of experience, psychopathology, and change is strikingly similar to Guidano's (1987) integration of cognitive therapy, attachment theory, and cybernetics, as well as to Wachtel's (1977; Gold & Wachtel, 1993) cyclical psychodynamics and to Andrews's (1993) active self theory and therapy. Guidano's (1991) approach aims at changing emotional experience and its underlying schematic organizers by repeatedly reviewing the patient's developmental history, and by observing and confronting how the patient regressively and redundantly structures experience, in the here and now with the therapist, as a repetition of that history. Guidano suggested that it is the therapist's job to disrupt the process of repetition by disengaging and by interacting with the patient in novel, emotionally charged ways. This interaction arouses, disconfirms, and provokes the building of new and more adaptive emotional organizing principles. Cyclical psychodynamically based integrative therapy, therapy based on the active self model, and other integrative systems that include a significant contribution from psychodynamic and cognitive-behavioral systems are oriented toward interventions that change the interpersonal and intrapsychic antecedents and reinforcers of problematic emotions, rather than toward the expansion of experience in itself. The causes or stimuli of emotions include interpersonal engagement, unconscious motives, conflicts, and deficits, or conscious ideas, perceptions, and fantasies. Reinforcing consequences include responses by others to emotional expression or avoidance. Certain intrapsychic states and reactions, including especially anxiety and subsequent defense mechanisms and interpersonal security operations, are highly reinforcing of emotional restriction. Their effectiveness in reducing anxiety is perhaps the most powerful reason to block the flow of experience that may be identified clinically. The expansion-of-consciousness experience is, in these integrative therapies, a welcome but not directly sought-after resultant of successful intervention.

A small number of integrative models that have been developed in work with severe personality disorders (Gold, 1990a, b; Gold & Stricker, 1993; Linehan, 1993) are concerned with building up or repairing experiential skill deficits and the underlying intrapsychic structural limitations that cause these dysfunctions. These deficits include weaknesses in the capacity to represent, bear, or modulate emotional experience and are treated with cognitive, behavioral, and imagery-based exercises that not only give rise to new skills and capacities but also aim to promote the internalization of new structures, schemas, and self- and object representations.

A SYNTHESIS OF INTEGRATIVE APPROACHES

The integrative therapies just discussed make a powerful and important contribution to theory and practice in psychotherapy integration because of their emphasis on affective and experiential issues, and particularly because of their accentuation of the clinical utility and significance of the patient's momentary, conscious experiencing. There is a bias among the majority of contributors to the literature in psychotherapy integration toward studying and working clinically with behavioral, cognitive, and psychodynamic (unconscious) variables. This bias makes descriptions of clinical practice experience distant and suggests that the patient's phenomenology, feelings, and bodily awareness are secondary epiphenomena that do not demand or deserve immediate or direct attention. However, as important as these client-centered and experientially based integrative works are, they may also be guilty of oversimplification or of too narrow a range of study.

The view of emotion and experience presented thus far in this chapter by integrative therapists centers on the process of feeling and experiencing and takes as an organizing factor the adaptive, motivational, and information-processing roles and functions of feelings, sensations, felt meanings, and affects. What is left out to some degree are the structural, developmental, and psychodynamic factors that govern emotional life, and that make experience tolerable, representable, and able to be processed and formulated in a socially acceptable and modulated way. Emotions and spontaneous experience form and are formed by unconscious and conscious motivational conflicts, interpersonal perceptions and interaction, and cognitively based information processing. Similarly, the intrapersonal and interactional behaviors and cognitive skills that are necessary to engage one's experience, to put it into words, and to act adaptively also receive less scrutiny in the models discussed above. The reason may be the philosophical and theoretical biases of the humanistic and experiential therapists, who are often loathe to include an account of structural factors or adaptive abilities (also known as *ego functions*). However, this omission may also be due to the clinical populations and clinical settings with whom and in which these theories and methods were worked out. Many of the therapists whose contributions were highlighted in this chapter's previous section have worked in research, university, or private practice settings, with an attendant increase in the proportion of higher functioning and more adaptively skilled patients, many of whom may come to therapy because of blocks or inhibitions in their ability to feel and to process experience fully. Clinicians of an integrative bent, who work more frequently with more disturbed patients (e.g., Gold, 1990a, b; Gold & Stricker, 1993; Hellcamp, 1993; Linehan, 1993), often add to such a focus on inhibitions of experience and affect a stress on issues of emotional dyscontrol, on the lack of affect tolerance and delay of gratification, or on other experiential difficulties that reflect unconscious deficits in personality structure and skill deficits in the cognitive and behavioral realms. Any fully integrative clinical approach to experiential and emotional distress must take into account all of these facets and variables in formulating treatment guidelines.

This embeddedness of emotional experience and the flow of awareness in a psychodynamic, cognitive, and interpersonal-action matrix suggests that a fully integrated therapy must include a careful consideration of the time and place for experientially or emotionally oriented interventions as well as make use of a variety of interventions as the need arises. The framework for integrated clinical decision making and intervention follows from the therapeutic stance of directed inquiry described in Chapter 4 and then relies on the presence of certain emotional and experiential markers. These markers may be decoded or deconstructed to yield inferences about the nature of the experiential task at hand.

Directed Inquiry as a Source of Experiential Exploration

As patients begin a guided review of any and all facets of their experience, behavior, and relationships, they become both more and less discomfited and anxious. Their anxiety decreases to the extent that they are able to perceive the therapist as the actively empathic, accepting ally that the therapist strives to be.

The narrative sources of anxiety and other dysphoria that are stimulated in the therapeutic relationship have already been considered in Chapter 2. Anxiety and other uncomfortable internal events produce in all patients their individual defenses, their ways of avoiding, distorting, or limiting emotions and awareness. Sometimes patients demonstrate difficulties in tolerating experiences and tendencies to react in explosive or exaggerated ways, or they invoke complementary reactions in the therapist that reinforce these alterations of feeling (the hooking mentioned by Reeve et al., 1993, or the interpersonal vicious circle cited by Wachtel, 1977). As patients discuss their experiences and events in their lives that occur outside the sessions, their reporting is also marked by gaps, omissions, and experiences about which they are confused, troubled, or pained (the problematic reaction marker mentioned by Rice, 1984, and Rice & Greenberg, 1991). Other experiences are mentioned matter-of-factly but are perceived by the therapist as problematic and as indicative of an experiential problem. Such a lack of reflectiveness resembles what Safran and Segal (1990) called an "embedded marker" and what Bohart (1990) discussed as a failure of corrective self evaluation. These markers point to two coincident problems. The first is the patient's reaction itself, and the second is the concrete or unreflective attitude that she or he holds with regard to that experience.

Experiential Markers and Integrative Clinical Decisions

As data are collected and experiential markers are noted in the relationship and in the larger life of the patient, the therapist is faced with several clinical problems and decision points. She or he must decide to intervene directly in experiential difficulties (à la Greenberg or Bohart) or to consider difficulties with emotions and consciousness derivatives of other processes that require immediate attention. Similarly, a choice must be made with regard to relationship-oriented interventions (Safran's unhooking and metacommunication) or interventions oriented toward intrapersonal or action issues that occur outside the sessions. These somewhat impossible choices and decisions may be guided in an immensely helpful way by the nature and type of marker felt and perceived by the therapist.

Markers that are conscious to both patient and therapist in an immediate and vivid sense are highly salient clinically and can be focused on profitably without fear of overlooking some other experience. The type of intervention to be used most often is readily suggested by the specifics of that marker. For example, when patient and therapist have become aware of some difficulty in their interaction, the process of unhooking and metacommunication has already begun. Such discussions may lead to enhanced awareness on the patient's part, or to the discovery of an underlying emotional, cognitive, or dynamic issue that may require a corresponding technique (a Gestalt exercise, cognitive restructuring, or interpretation, respectively). In like vein, the report of a troubling or confusing problematic reaction marker or vulnerability marker leads easily to the Rice and Greenberg (1991) techniques of experiential search and emotional prizing as the interventions of first choice.

When embedded markers are noticed by the therapist, she or he must consider the locus of the lack of awareness (outside or inside the sessions), the nature of the unnoticed experiential difficulty (e.g., overreaction, lack of control and tolerance, or emotional inhibition or repression) and the source of the patient's incapacity for self-evaluation and reflection (e.g., the operation of unconscious defenses, a lack of skill based on structural deficits, cognitive limitations, or interpersonal dynamics). While maintaining a sense of respect and positive regard for the patient, the therapist must take an active and confrontational role in pointing out both the experiential problem and the patient's lack of awareness of that problem. When and if the patient is able to accept both of these observations, other interventive choices must be considered. Often the immediate task is working with the patient's shame, anger, or hurt at being made aware of such an oversight or blindness on his or her part in relation to his or her own flow of awareness. These reactions can be resolved through a combination of a cognitive review of the negative thoughts and attitudes evoked by the confrontation and, if necessary, a dynamic interpretation of the underlying issues of self-punitiveness or the need for perfection, control, and mastery, among others.

When the patient is ready to consider both his or her difficulties in experiencing and the embedded marker which brought this issue to the therapist's attention, many techniques may be appropriate. Issues of underreaction and emotional inhibition may be most responsive to the active Gestalt exercises favored by Greenberg et al. (1993) and by focal expressive therapists. These techniques, if successful, not only aid the patient in integrating and accepting experiences but bring into consciousness the object representation and the cognitive-emotional schemas and historical issues that structure such inhibition. Such active work in arousing and integrating emotions is most often effective with the overcontrolled patient who demonstrates an isolating and intellectualizing defense. Dynamic and cognitive work is too easily assimilated into these patients' existing character structures and methods of limiting experience (Andrews, 1993; Beutler & Hodgson, 1993). Patients who have repressive defensives or who are somehow able to totally exclude entire aspects of their emotional life from awareness sometimes benefit from preliminary interpretive work in order to identify potential affects and feeling states that may be aimed at in experiential exercises. Interpretive work is also crucial when emotional limitations are the outcome of repressed or dissociated conflicts between sets of emotional rules or schemas. Sometimes, patients cannot utilize an experiential search, a focusing exercise, or a here-and-now intervention until their unconscious attachments to their experiential limitations (identifications with parental figures and their experiential modes) are explored and resolved.

Emotional overreaction and loss of control, as well as the related problems of a lack of affect tolerance and an inability to delay action, seem to respond most effectively to interventions that build new cognitive and behavioral skills and at the same time repair deficits in the underlying unconscious representational structures (Gold, 1990a, b; Gold & Stricker, 1993; Linehan, 1993). These problems can be helped by teaching soothing self-talk and self-statements, comforting imagery, self-talk and imagery that guide the person through ideational solutions to problems in place of action, social skills training, and other related behavioral methods. In addition to providing a habilitative cognitive process, active learning and therapeutic instruction in managing experience give the patient an immediate sense of mastery and competence. Out of repeated feelings of being capable and whole may develop a more congruent and complete sense of the self, and more benign and reliable representations of others may be internalized as the interaction with the therapist is processed and stored in emotional memory (Gold, 1990b).

The failure in self-corrective evaluation and in experiential flow that typifies an embedded marker is sometimes overcome by the work described above. At other points, as Bohart (1990, 1992) has suggested, direct instruction or intervention in this process is required. This may take the form of cognitive exercises in self-monitoring, keeping a log of dreams or symptoms, freewriting of experiences, and Gestalt work aimed at enhancing the momentary awareness of bodily and psychic states, among other. Enhanced self-reflection is often a goal of interpretive work aimed at resolving unconscious conflicts that result in a concrete defensive orientation to life. The empathic metacommunication of hooks, patterns of engagement, and covert ways of involving the therapist as a pathogenic accomplice often leads to disconfirmation of transference expectations that reflect feared consequences of open emotionality (Andrews, 1993; Gold & Wachtel, 1993; Reeve et al., 1993; Safran & Segal, 1990; Wachtel, 1977). Identification with the therapist's ability to be aware of, reflective of, and comfortable with emotional expression is a powerful vehicle for change as new modes of processing experience are internalized just after old emotional schemas and structures have been neutralized, disconfirmed, and abandoned through novel experiences in and out of the therapeutic interaction.

NARRATIVE AND EXPERIENCE

Try to imagine your favorite song stripped of its musical track, sung only in *a cappella* form. Or consider an action or horror movie without a sound track, *Swan Lake* danced to silence, or a radio broadcast of a baseball or football game without the sound of the crowd. What would your experience be of a glass of fine wine if it were as colorless as spring water, even if the taste were retained. What would a Thanksgiving meal be like if there were no anticipatory odors and sounds to precede the actual consumption of the meal. Finally, try to imagine the reduced impact of an Impressionist painting if the colors were removed.

The impact of many of life's experiences and the effect of many narrative units are not conveyed in linear, verbal, and linguistically encoded ways. In all of the examples above, I have jettisoned the stimuli that most of us would equate with emotion: the parts of the event that move us, affect us directly in our sensory and bodily existence, and tell us immediately about how we are being affected, and about what is yet to come. The telling of stories is often intended to move us viscerally as well as to impart information. Otherwise, why would we need adjectives and adverbs? Why would writers spend so much time in describing characters, geography, interiors, and other elements of the story that are not essential to the plot? The ability of human beings to enjoy the repetition of stories, the outcomes of which are known, points to the central role of the generation of emotion in narration: We listen again and again because we desire the emotional experience that accompanies the telling of the tale.

This immediate visceral function of the narrative is, as discussed above, highly informative and evolutionarily protective. How we feel, how our bodies react, and our immediate sensory "take" on an experience orient us rapidly, automatically, and often more accurately than the linear, linguistically derived orientation that accrues from cognitive processing. Emotions are the backdrop of the narrative. They foreshadow, accompany, and deepen the meaning of an event and they linger after the thought has departed. As in music, art, or cooking, the linear and the immediate must exist in some sort of dialectical relationship. The role and place of emotion in a healthy narrative are in constant flux. At times, cognitive processing and action take precedence, and we feel only later. At other stages, emotion should be in the foreground and can be fit with words only after some time and effort.

Within any song, the words and the music may complement each other or may be out of balance. Just as the work of the Beatles (or Pearl Jam or Cole Porter) would have less impact without the musical tracks, the meaning and effect would be altered significantly if the vocals were missing or were drowned out by the bass and drums. A movie soundtrack may underscore the action or may contradict what is happening in some jarring way. Certain modern paintings are notable for the contradictions between their morbid subject matter and their bright hues. A psychological narrative may be notable for the imbalance between affect and information: Emotion may be missing at key moments, may be subdued or inhibited in a consistent and chronic way, or may occur in exaggerated bursts that interfere with the story rather than guiding it. Another narrative dysfunction of emotion includes those parts of the story wherein the verbal and the felt contradict each other, leaving the person with two simultaneous plots to follow. Finally, the narratives of many patients contain specific story lines about emotional experience in general or about discrete emotions in specific: Anger may be forbidden because of its perceived effect on one's parents, love may be construed as necessary at all costs, sadness may be written in as safer than joy, and so on. These emotional subplots may be conscious or unconscious, but their impact is usually very obvious in the patient's descriptions of his or her life, and in the interaction with the therapist.

As the patient's narrative is understood, the healthy and pathogenic ways in which emotional experience is integrated become prominent. The markers of difficulty of emotional processing that were discussed in the last section of this chapter are also indicators of narrative dysfunction. The techniques that are prescribed by those markers will lead, if successful, to changes in the person's narrative: The colors will be highlighted, deleted, or muted into more becoming shades; the volume on the soundtrack will be adjusted; and so forth. A change in narrative can and often does lead to changes in the person's ability to feel freely, to modulate emotions that were excessively strong or harsh, or to balance cognitive and emotional processing sequentially and simultaneously. Correspondingly, change in accessing emotional experience can and does lead to important and deep narrative revision: As a person can feel more broadly, more extensively, and in a more nuanced way, his or her adaptive resources grow. That person is no longer limited to one aspect of life, and his or her appreciation of the affective side of life is incorporated into representations of the self, of relationships, and of possibilities for engaging the world. Discovering or changing the capacity for joy, sadness, rage, lust, fear, or any other emotion can and does cause a reconsideration of the identity one has constructed, the roles one takes and gives to others, and the acceptability of interactions that are emotionally arousing.

Psychotherapy that is guided by this narrative perspective thus utilizes experiential interventions both to modify emotional processing and to use experiential change to correct the person's dysfunctional tale. Additionally, active intervention in behavior and cognition, as well as psychodynamic interventions, is used before, concurrently with, and after an experiential task. These techniques are required when the person cannot access some emotional state without changing a way of thinking or behaving, or when unconscious conflict leads to defenses that are aimed at the inhibition of emotion. An example would be someone whose lack of sexual desire has led to a total avoidance of potential partners for fear of shame and failure. Behavioral and cognitive work aimed at building self-confidence and at social assertion may precede and accompany experiential exploration, as would interpretation if the patient's report indicated the need.

CLINICAL EXAMPLE: JAMES

As James's history and daily life unfolded and were explored in therapy, it became apparent to him and to therapist that he was able to experience anxiety, worry, and depression frequently and severely but otherwise was relatively affectless and dissociated from bodily experience, and particularly from pleasure of any sort. His oft-repeated description of himself as a "writing machine" demonstrated a magnificent intellect, which also dominated his interactions with himself and the world. Also emergent in the therapeutic relationship, but not in James's consciousness, was his factual, knowledge-based approach to all interpersonal relatedness, as well as a kind of smug amusement and enjoyment connected to his discussions of his emotionless and anhedonic life. It was clear that the emotional sound track to his life story had been omitted almost entirely, with the exception of the occasional trumpet blares that signaled his fear and pain. As a result, James could not use emotional states to guide his behavior or to complete his construal of life. Additionally, and quite outside his awareness, his depictions of the interactions that could generate intimacy, warmth, and affection were phobic and terrible, casting such possibilities for contact with others as events to be shunned. Therefore, he had learned exquisitely effective ways of avoiding closeness and of devaluing it, and he had failed to learn the skills that would be necessary to establish intimate connections with other people.

These experiential issues were worked with in a number of ways. As past and present in James's life began to fit together, his anxieties, drivenness, and lack of emotional contact were understood and interpreted as unconscious identifications with facets of his parents' characters and the familial climate in which he had been reared. This process led not to an experiential or emotional change, but to a point of agreement between patient and therapist for further exploration. Further interpretive work, coupled with metacommunication and unhooking within the therapeutic relationship, led to deeper understanding of and to a change in the feeling tone about James's overt but unintegrated, smug amusement at his own pain. As he became more interested in and concerned about this issue, an experiential search was begun. This plunge into his flow of sensation and affect led to images and feelings that he noted had probably always been at the fringes of his awareness, but from which he had thus far recoiled in pain. These feelings included grief, bitterness, anger, shame, and self-blame connected to the rejections, abandonments, perversity, and apathetic lack of interest with which he remembered having been treated by both parents.

The experiential search was concluded with James's narrative about his development's having been shaken and disconfirmed to a considerable degree. However, he had a great deal of difficulty in focusing on the experiences, feelings, and memories that had been elicited, chiefly because of the shame, embarrassment, and anxiety he felt in being open emotionally with another person. Most important, his intellectualized character style and unconscious, phobic construal of emotions worked to keep these new depictions of himself from being fully integrated into his self-image. As we noted in the last chapter, Gestalt exercises, in which he engaged in dialogues with his parents, were experienced as so powerful in an immediate way that James was then able to make these narrative accommodations. Following these interventions, these reactive emotions and their new place in his story were explored via interpretation of their roots, again in his identifications with certain features of his father's character, and also through cognitive and behavioral exercises aimed at the gradual exposure and revelation of such inner affective states. These efforts yielded a surprising sense of sadness and pain, which once again was subjected to an experiential search. This process eventuated in James's openness to a deep sense of emptiness, deprivation, and anger, as he suggested, "I feel that if I were to give up my fears about being emotional, I would give up the only things I ever learned or got from my father. That's the emptiness, and I'm furious at him, though I can't hold onto it." Discussions of this type suggested that work with unfinished business through active techniques would be helpful, as did the powerful intellectualizing and isolating defenses that James used, which made interpretation and cognitive work only dimly effective on an experiential level.

James was encouraged to work with his feelings about his father in a two-chair, present-oriented vocal dialogue with that parent. He found this task difficult, both because of its unfamiliarity and because he felt he did not have the inner strength to bear and to control his anger and sadness. Here, imagery of a self-soothing sort was employed, as were self-soothing cognitive experiments. The interaction between James and the therapist also came in for much attention during this period, as James attempted to engage the therapist in intellectual discussions, and his unconscious transferences were confronted, explored, and disconfirmed. This work led to James's spontaneous recognition and awkward but moving mention of the closeness he felt to the therapist, and to the novelty, pleasure, and terror he felt in being aware of those feelings and in admitting them openly.

Finally, James was able to proceed with the Gestalt exercises connected with his unfinished business with his father and, soon after, with his mother. As he did so, his capacity to feel angry, bitter, and sad increased enormously, at times, however, requiring more cognitive-behavioral work in affect-tolerance-building exercises and images. A long period followed of grief and mourning, which were met largely through empathic exploration in an emotionally prizing, positively charged interaction. During this period, James began to write and read about psychological and psychotherapeutic topics, an activity that he identified spontaneously as the building of an identification with the therapist and the therapist's modes of experiencing himself and the world.

During and following these gains, James began to become more concerned about his lack of satisfactions sexually and recreationally, and about his distance from his wife, children, and friends. He began to set behavioral and interactional goals for himself in which he would assign himself a certain number of interpersonal tasks that made him anxious, such as approaching his wife sexually, telling her or his children that he loved them, leaving work early to go to a movie or a ball game, or confronting his boss about an unfair assignment or rude behavior. As he moved through these interactions, both conscious and embedded markers of blocking and constriction of his ability to feel and to be open to himself were met with confrontations, interpretation, and active experiential exploration. This work coincided with periods of work on the therapeutic relationship, wherein, once again, James's intellectual methods of interaction would surface inevitably whenever he had moved toward a fear-or anxiety-provoking emotional experience.

In this last period of the treatment, the work in and outside the relationship evoked for James a deeply felt and experienced sense of the narrational rules he had established for himself in living and surviving in his family. He now believed that both parents had been deeply disturbed, incompetent, and enraged persons who had hidden these facets of themselves behind a facade of polite inaccessibility.

James was deeply moved by these perceptions and noted that he felt he had undergone some sort of internal revolution, which frightened him but which also allowed him to begin to work at a new set of construals and ideas that would coexist comfortably with his emerging capacity for experiential openness.

Active Interventions for Behavioral and Cognitive Change

TRADITIONAL THERAPEUTIC USES OF ACTIVE INTERVENTION

All psychotherapies are based on the processes of learning and directed behavioral change. However, the sectarian schools of traditional therapy differ considerably with regard to their emphases on these processes and the roles given to instruction and direction on the part of the therapist. Obviously, behavioral and cognitive therapies are the prototypes of active, directive, and didactic psychotherapy. From behavior therapy's earliest days, when its ideology flaunted its roots in the laboratory and in learning theory, until today, the behavior therapist has been considered an educator, a director, and a guide to change. Overt behavioral change is both the method and the goal of this therapy, and it is almost impossible to think of a behavioral intervention about which this point is not true. Pioneering behavioral techniques such as systematic desensitization (Wolpe, 1958) were introduced openly as action-based substitutes for the then-current methods (experiential and psychodynamic), which were not focused on immediate change. The ongoing testing and refinement of interventions that are derived from classical conditioning, operant conditioning, and social learning paradigms share this over riding concern (Glass & Arnkoff, 1992).

Goldfried (1991) identified the central change ingredient in behavior therapy as being the facilitation and provision of new experiences. These interactions with the environment provide the patient with the opportunity to learn new skills, to correct cognitive distortions, and to experience differently the self in action. In their review of the core assumptions of behavioral theories and methods, Fishman and Franks (1992) noted that these systems continue to place assisted learning by the patient at the center of the work. The therapist is active in manipulating the environment, in promoting exposure to feared stimuli and covert experience, and in demonstrating and teaching novel patterns of thinking and action.

The creators of cognitive and rational-emotive therapy were clear and explicit about their respective debts to the concepts and methods of behavior therapy, and each system describes the role of the therapist as directive, didactic, and concerned explicitly with change (Beck & Emory, 1985; Ellis, 1984). One of the unique contributions of cognitive psychotherapy has been its demonstration of the possibilities and advantages of intervening actively and directly in covert, intrapsychic processes. It is this feature that has perhaps led some (Alford & Norcross, 1991; Beck, 1991) to identify cognitive therapy as the prototypical integrative method.

Psychoanalysis and the humanistic psychotherapies might be located at one end of a continuum of therapist directiveness and educational activity, with the range of cognitive-behavioral therapies positioned at the other end of that line. These therapies also differ considerably with regard to the types of learning they favor, as well as the locus of the learning experiences that are deemed theoretically and clinically desirable.

Psychodynamic therapy and client-centered therapy, in their most pure or classical forms, share perhaps the most extreme distrust and disregard of active intervention in symptoms, dysfunctional behaviors, and cognitive difficulties. The arguments against an instructive interventive role, as well as the use of directed behavioral and ideational techniques offered by adherents to these two systems, overlap to some degree but are also made unique by the characteristics of the ideologies and methods of the two approaches. Dynamic and client-centered therapies are in agreement about the type and locus of advantageous therapeutic learning. The intrapersonal or intrapsychic processes of expanding awareness, or of developing insight into previously unconscious or unsymbolized aspects of experience, are the learning processes that are central to both types of therapy. An increased understanding of interpersonal events may be almost or equally important in certain variants of dynamic or client-centered therapy. Clearly, both give little emphasis to, or have little explicit regard for, the types of learning processes most dear to academic experimental psychologists, learning theorists, or cognitive-behavioral therapists. In fact, methods that enable patients to directly change behavior and thinking, to adapt to the environment more effectively, and efficiently and to unlearn or decrease the frequency of symptomatic behaviors and internal processes have traditionally been looked on as undesirable and countertherapeutic by many classical analysts and Rogerian therapists.

Psychoanalysts of most persuasions are concerned with behavior change and cognitive modification as by-products or derivatives of underlying shifts in unconscious motivational states and conflicts. In particular, classical dynamic theory states in no uncertain terms that significant symptomatic relief and functional change occurs only after insight, abreaction, and catharsis of previously repressed dynamic material have been established (Menniger, 1958). Therefore, the patient's thoughts, images, and reports of overt behavior are of use only to the extent that they can be vehicles of inference that lead to interpretation. Classical analytic thinking posits that directive activity on the part of the analyst muddies and obscures the free flow of associations on the part of the patient and makes interpretations invalid and perhaps even harmful. While symptomatic relief through advice, hypnosis, and other rational and educative methods may be possible, such interventions are thought to be parameters that place limits on a successful analysis (Eissler, 1953) by making unconscious material totally inaccessible to interpretation. Other unwanted effects of directive work may be a flight into health or premature termination due to rapid symptom relief, or difficult complications in the therapeutic alliance and transference relationship that will not yield easily to interpretation.

As dynamic therapists have become more interested in problems of character disorder (Reich, 1949), interpersonal and object relationships (Mitchell, 1988; Sullivan, 1953), and cognitive and perceptual structure and style (Klein, 1971; Shapiro, 1965), dynamic theory and therapy have yielded more of a clinically relevant position to the patient's behavior, thought processes, and adaptive capacities and strategies. However, while the data set has been expanded, the type and number of useful techniques have not kept pace. Added to interpretation have been the methods of confrontation (the pointing out of a behavioral or cognitive event) and clarification (the exploration of the antecedents, correlates, consequences, and conscious meanings of that thought or action). These techniques are generally considered preparatory to the interpretation of the unconscious conflicts and historical precursors of the action.

Certain dynamic therapists have taken a maverick position with regard to the use of directive and educative techniques in psychodynamic therapies. Perhaps the first of these clinicians was Freud himself, who in an early paper of psychoanalytic technique (1912) pointed out that some phobic patients needed to be compelled by the analyst to face the object of their fears for analytic progress to occur. Freud (1909) also saw that certain obsessive-compulsive patients had to be encouraged or required to give up their rituals and compulsions. These actions on the part of the analyst were necessary in order to resolve and overcome the defensive, resistant aspect of the phobic avoidances and compulsive behavior. Freud understood that unless these behaviors were altered, insight and catharsis would be absent or severely limited.

While most subsequent analytic work ignored Freud's suggestions, Alexander and French (1946) boldly expanded his suggestions. They argued that insight is often a consequence of behavioral and attitudinal change, rather than always being the cause of change. As a result, they developed a modified and active psychodynamic therapy in which the actions of the therapist are geared toward inducing new behaviors and emotional experiences in and for the patient (the "corrective emotional experience") in combination with the traditional work of interpretation. The work of Alexander and French is frequently cited by psychodynamically oriented students of psychotherapy integration.

Client-centered therapy would cease to be client-centered if its practice were expanded to include directive interventions of a behavioral or cognitive nature. The requisite unconditional positive regard and empathy that are the relational foundation of this approach are violated to an extreme degree by an attitude of instruction and correction, which Rogers and other client-centered purists would probably argue rest on an assumption of expertise and superior knowledge about the patient's experience. Since the therapist cannot know more about the person's phenomenology, experiences, and choices than that person does at that moment, such expertise is fallacious and may reflect the therapist's own state of incongruence. As noted above, any intervention that changes the work of the therapy from an exploration of the nuances of subjectivity to a discussion of overt acts as an end in itself is entirely antithetical to the spirit and method of a truly Rogerian model of client-centered work.

Other models of humanistic therapy allow for a certain level of instruction, education, and directed work. The Gestalt therapist works in a very active and directive manner in confronting resistances and blocks in awareness. He or she requests that the patient attend to some aspect of his or her posture, vocal tone, facial expression, movement, choice of words, or other communicative gesture or experience. In pursuit of change, a Gestalt therapist actively suggests experiments and exercises that are aimed at overcoming or undoing the previously identified experiential blockages. However, where this therapy differs in a highly significant way from the educative approaches embodied by cognitive-behavioral therapy is in the goals of directive intervention. Symptoms and behavior patterns are of concern to the Gestalt therapist to the extent that these problems signify an inauthentic way of life and a person whose awareness of needs and situations is constricted or is distorted. Changes in behavior and cognition are valuable if they lead to an expanded and articulated awareness. Also, and most important, Gestalt exercises do not prescribe or instruct directly in terms of suggesting new behaviors or ways of processing information. Rather, they lead to change by heightening the person's awareness of conflictual needs and inner states, and by increasing tension until blocks are undone. The Gestalt therapist works from a theory or methodology that suggests that old habits need to be undone not gradually and through learning principles, but through a process of intense and immediate emotional relearning. (See the following chapter for more detail on Gestalt interventions.)

Existential therapists do not often engage in directive intervention but rely heavily on confrontation and exploration of behavior to understand its meanings and its place in the patient's existence (Bugenthal & Kleiner, 1993; May & Yalom, 1989). However, there is one significant exception to this statement, and that is found in the work of Frankl (1960), who developed the existential system that he called "logotherapy." Truly an existentialist, Frankl maintained that the search for meaning was the central motivational issue in human life, and that psychopathology expressed a loss or a breakdown of a connection to meaning. In order to demonstrate to patients the workings and existential impact of dysfunctional behavior and symptoms, Frankl utilized certain active techniques, including especially paradoxical methods and the prescription of symptoms and problematic behaviors. His goal was not symptomatic improvement or new learning, though such changes often occurred. Rather, in demonstrations to patients that their alien and seemingly uncontrollable experiences and acts could be effected volitionally and consciously, the meaning of these behaviors and the willful, deliberate meanings and desires embodied in them became apparent to the patient. With this recovery of authentic meaning, the will of the patient was liberated and expanded, and more authentic choices became possible.

INTEGRATIVE APPROACHES TO THE USE OF ACTION-ORIENTED INTERVENTIONS

There are two broad classes of action-oriented, integrative interventive approaches. The first may be called *prescriptive*, in that techniques are chosen from the perspective of finding the best match for a particular symptom, behavior pattern, or cognitive dysfunction. The techniques are used in pure forms as they are described in the original cognitive-behavioral literature, and their clinical aims and goals are traditional and focused as well. Some of the matching or prescription of technique to symptom is based on clinical intuition and experience, while in some of these integrative approaches there is an attempt to turn, as frequently as is possible, to the empirical literature in psychotherapy for guidance.

The second class of action-oriented interventions groups together those approaches that aim at deep and complex representational, psychodynamic, and structural changes through behavioral, cognitive, and interpersonal methods. These approaches are part of systems that aim at a theoretical integration of psychotherapy as well as at the integration of technical procedures (see Chapters 1 and 2). Such methods are selected not only because of their effects on a focal symptom or action, but because of their inferred and desired impact on other spheres and levels of functioning. The interventions selected are sometimes standard behavioral and cognitive techniques, such as desensitization, self-monitoring, or assertiveness training. These methods are used because they yield the expectable, standard therapeutic effect action or thought. In addition, these gains influence patients' perceptions of themselves or of others or enable them to face and become aware of some of the unconscious factors that were hidden in and behind an ideational or behavioral problem, to name just two possibilities. Other action-oriented interventions are more original and comprise what Wachtel (1991) called "seamless" integration. This terms refers to techniques that are formed of an integrated set of principles and goals. For example, the behavioral procedures of response prevention and exposure can be combined with interpretation. This integrative event occurs when an interpretation is offered that is based on wording that provides insight into unconscious processes and at the same time lessens the likelihood that the patient will avoid the anxiety connected with this new awareness (Wachtel, 1993).

Focal and Prescriptive Uses of Action-Oriented Interventions

Lazarus's (1992) multimodal therapy, Beutler's (Beutler & Hodgson, 1993) prescriptive psychotherapy or systematic eclectic psychotherapy (Beutler & Consoli, 1992), and the common-factors eclectic therapy of Garfield (1992) are among the most widely cited and influential integrative systems that rely on prescriptive matching of intervention to a focal behavior or problem. The prescription of a therapeutic method is based on a careful and individualized assessment along many different dimensions, and it is the configuration of such profiles that most clearly differentiates these approaches. These therapists share a repertoire that includes a wide range of cognitive, behavioral, interpersonal, and experiential techniques. They differ most clearly in their decision-making concepts and methods.

Lazarus's (1992) approach relies on his assessment of the firing order within first, second, and subsequent levels of the BASIC ID profile (see Chapter 1 for details of this profile). As the interrelationships between strengths, deficits, excesses, and deviant aspects of functioning in each mode of the profile become apparent, the therapist selects the appropriate points of intervention. Lazarus (1989) emphasized clearly his preference for empirically tested methods and was especially disdainful of psychodynamic methods and of efforts at theoretical integration. Lazarus (1992) presented a guide for the prescription of certain types of change mechanisms and interventions for problems in each of the modes of the BASIC ID profile. Problems in *behavior* respond to contingency control and operant techniques. Abreactive techniques and emotional acceptance methods are suited to work in the *affect* mode, while *sensory* difficulties respond best to methods focused on tension release and reduction and on anhedonic enhancement. Lazarus prescribed positive and coping self-imagery for the *imagery* mode, as well as some of the standard methods of thought restructuring for pathology in *cognition*. Finally, *interpersonal relationships* are treated with modeling and the management of unhealthy input from others, while *drugs/biology* problems may require substance abuse interventions, psychotropic medication, or improvement in exercise and nutrition.

Beutler's prescriptive psychotherapy (Beutler & Consoli, 1992; Beutler & Hodgson, 1993) orders the use of directive and behavioral methods when its exhaustive assessment of patient, therapist, and situational characteristics yields a particular matching profile. This profile is based on the research literature that is concerned with finding the best fit between patient, therapist, and intervention. Beutler and Hodgson (1993) suggested that directive interventions are most likely to be useful with patients who do not experience a loss of autonomy and control when such methods are used. Behavioral methods such as modeling, reinforcement, and social skills training are also favored with patients whose conduct is marked by a lack of control or adaptive skill, and whose defenses and coping strategies tend toward projection and externalization. Cognitive interventions are best matched to clients who are troubled by subjectively distressing and overly powerful feelings of depression, rage and anger, or anxiety, and who are capable of reviewing their self-talk and their distressing ideational patterns.

Garfield (1992) organized his system of eclectic psychotherapy around the common-factors approach to integration (see Chapter 1). Among the common factors that Garfield stressed are the change mechanisms of reinforcement, the provision of new information and skills, the confrontation of feared situations and inner experiences, and the extinction of conditioned anxiety. He does not work out of as formal a prescriptive model as do the therapists just described, for he believes that technical decisions should be guided by the patient's perceptions of her or his needs, goals, and priorities. When a problem has been selected for intervention, Garfield's approach matches the desired outcome to one of the common change mechanisms listed above. The final step is the choice of an empirically validated intervention that has been demonstrated to yield the wished-for results.

USING ACTION-ORIENTED METHODS TO PROMOTE STRUCTURAL, DYNAMIC, AND REPRESENTATIONAL CHANGE

Directive and behavioral interventions are used within several systems of psychotherapy integration that share certain important theoretical and clinical components. These systems are all efforts at integration at a theoretical level and contain explicit theories of personality and of psychopathology out of which their technical integrations and innovations proceed (see Chapters 1 and 2). There are two loose subgroups within this class. In one, the organizing personality theory is intrapsychic, though not necessarily psychodynamic. Didactic and directive methods in these systems aim at reaching and modifying intrapersonal processes while first or concurrently altering symptomatic behavior and ideation. Quite often, the active interventions are aimed at internally generated anxiety its sequelae, including defense mechanisms and other intrapsychic responses that inhibit new experience, awareness, and behavioral change. Change is thus understood to be multidirectional, and in their broad range, intrapsychic and behavioral processes are understood to be mutually influential, at all levels of awareness.

An interactional and contextual view of personality is shared by the integrative therapists in the second subgroup. This view encompasses the ideas of the position just described but adds to it the awareness of the impact of current interactions with other persons on the maintenance of intrapsychic variables, personality structure, cognitive style and content, overt behavior and psychopathology. The collection of personality theories represented here might invoke the metaphor of the circle to describe the feedforward, feedback, and homeostatic interaction between intrapersonal issues and interpersonal events. Active interventions may be and are employed in these models at any point on the circle: to produce direct change in behavior thought, or mode of relatedness, and also to intervene indirectly in the dynamic, representational, and structural issues that shape and are shaped by these observable actions.

The two subgroups share a multidirectional view of the relationship between insight and change that, as noted earlier, was perhaps introduced by Alexander and French (1946). Change sometimes precedes and brings about insight in the form of new conscious contents, and at other times, making an unconscious issue accessible to awareness is a necessary precondition for new behavior and experience.

ACTIVE INTERVENTION IN INTRAPSYCHIC PROCESSES

Fensterheim (1993) organized his system of behavioral psychotherapy around a detailed behavioral assessment, which leads into standard behavioral interventions. Interventions such as relaxation, desensitization, and imagery satiation usually produce the desired and sufficient behavioral change. Additionally, Fensterheim has been able to adapt these active methods to the aim of intervening at the psychodynamic levels of the person's functioning (Level 3 in his system) and at the interfacing level of functioning that is the locus of both behaviorally mediated and dynamically involved symptoms and resistances. In Fensterheim's view, intrapsychic and interpersonal defenses can be resolved through the use of behavioral methods such as desensitization and imagery-based satiation. Here, the therapist moves to formulations drawn from Levels 2 and 3 and guides the content of the behavioral work on the basis of those additional assessments. She or he assumes that defenses are prompted by anxiety generated by unconscious childhood memories and associated motives that the patient chooses to avoid in order to reduce the conscious experience of anxiety. Once such memories are inferred from the patient's thoughts about a certain symptom or behavior problem, he or she can be exposed gradually in imagery to related content until the associated anxieties are reduced. Once this is accomplished, the defenses are no longer necessary, and the basic psychodynamic issues may emerge spontaneously. This method is utilized when standard behavioral work is met with obstacles, which indicate a need for further assessment and intervention.

This synthesis of behavioral methods and psychodynamic content is very nearly identical to two pioneering systems of psychotherapy integration: the psychodynamic behavior therapy introduced by Feather and Rhodes (1972a, b), and implosion therapy, conceptualized by Stampfl and Levis (1967) as a learning-theory-based method for deconditioning the patient to the unconscious effects of early trauma. Both of these therapies rely on basic exposure techniques that are adapted, à la Fensterheim, to produce extinction of the conditioned association of memories and repressed experiences with anxiety. Feather and Rhoades made extensive use of systematic desensitization in which the patient went through a hierarchy of symbolic scenes that moved toward a feared or avoided unconscious conflict. Implosion therapy favors a highly concentrated exposure to such material in the manner of the behavioral technique of flooding. In each case, we observe action and directive work being utilized to produce changes in unconscious processes of defense and avoidance, with the hoped-for results of lessened anxiety that is followed by symptom reduction. Insight and the awareness of repressed material are often a by-product of these therapies as well.

Wolfe's (1992a, b) treatment of anxiety and phobic disorders proceeds from the theoretical integration of cognitive and learning principles, psychodynamic concepts, and existential ideas. He presented a theory of the anxiety disorders that is based on the tacit presence of catastrophic imagery of an existential sort. In his view, underlying the patient's fear of physical harm and dangers are concerns about such experiences as merging, humiliation and shame, and abandonment, and about conflicts over such issues as autonomy and dependency and the limits of one's capabilities. His approach utilizes a sequence of imagery, behavioral, cognitive, and experiential techniques to provide symptomatic relief and, more important, to provide an opportunity for change at "deeper" levels of self-experience and unconscious conflict. Imagery techniques are used to elicit the tacit catastrophic ideas. Relaxation and anxiety-management procedures, including deep breathing, decatastrophizing thinking, and didactic instruction about anxiety, enable the patient to tolerate his or her distress.

Once the patient has identified and better tolerated the tacit conflicts and existential issues, a phase of conflict resolution begins. Conflicts are met with modified two-chair Gestalt exercises in which the two sides of the conflict are embodied, a dialogue is established, and then concrete behavioral steps are decided on and are tested as a way of moving toward some synthesis of the covert struggle. These active methods lead to change in emotional processing, self-experience, and the representational schemas that mediate the patient's adaptation.

Wolfe's amalgam of behavioral, existential, cognitive, and dynamic constructs and methods is highly similar to my description of a theoretically integrated therapy for anxiety (Gold, 1993a). However, my work relies more heavily on in vivo exposure techniques for symptomatic relief and for access to underlying conflicts, in ways that resemble the use of behavioral methods by Fensterheim, Feather and Rhodes, and Stampfl and Levis. Also, in the stage of conflict resolution, I view interpretation and active enactment in the therapeutic relationship of faulty attachment experiences as critical sources of change in deeper structures of self- and object representations. This treatment for anxiety also provides corrective experiences through imagery and cognitive skill building that are aimed at providing the patient with the raw data out of which to form adaptive images of the self and others.

The extensive interest in treating borderline and narcissistic disorders has given rise to many therapeutic innovations, including a number of theoretical integrations of psychotherapies. These integrative therapies share a concern with the deficits in internal structure, object and self-representations, and the ability to assimilate and handle emotional experience that are demonstrated by these patients. Each integrative system uses cognitive, behavioral, and instructional methods in synthetic ways, guided by the specifics of the deficit or unconscious issue at hand, to repair or modify these underlying weaknesses.

Linehan's (1993) dialectical behavior therapy is based on a theoretical integration of behavioral, cognitive, interpersonal, emotional, and biological factors. Borderline disorders are thought to develop in physiologically vulnerable persons who are reared in an invalidating environment. This vulnerability is a hypersensitivity to stimuli and a relative lack of emotional regulation ability; the invalidating experiences are those in which significant others fail to respond accurately and empathically to inner emotional states. The interaction of these two factors eventuates in a person who exists in a state of chronic emotional vulnerability and dyscontrol, with a corresponding internal representation of the self at risk to invalidating others.

Heard and Linehan (1994) based their therapy on the dialectical tug between providing an accepting, validating experience for the patient and the need to provide new learning experiences. These educative measures include teaching problem-solving skills through modeling, communication training, assertiveness training, contingency management, cognitive restructuring, and exposure. Of much importance is the teaching of distress tolerance and of emotional regulation skills, as these address the basic deficit in the patient's pathology. The combination of such learning and change in the context of validation promotes restructuring of the basic emotional and biological vulnerabilities. Weston (1988) and others (Gold, 1990a, b; Gold & Stricker, 1993; Hellcamp, 1993) have targeted the structural and representational deficits in borderline and narcissistic disorders for intervention with cognitive and imagery-based techniques. These writers have argued that such active methods can be designed to correct behavioral and cognitive dysfunctions and, at the same time, foster the internalization of new views of the self in relation to others. These modified interventions teach the patient a new form of self and object relatedness as they correct an overt symptom or inhibition.

ACTIVE INTERVENTION IN CONTEXTUAL
THEORETICAL INTEGRATION

Those integrative systems that are based on circular, contextual theories of personality share certain significant ways of utilizing active interventions. The purposes and goals of these methods are also held in common. Behavioral, cognitive, and systemic techniques are employed to change their typically targeted functions, as in the traditional therapies from which they are drawn. As in the integrative systems that are intrapsychic in nature, active techniques are used to modify and to habilitate underlying schemas, object and self-representations, and psychodynamic conflict. The unique contribution of these contextual approaches to the integrative application of active methods is the use of such methods in an interpersonal context.

The clinical application of these interventions is driven by theories posit an inextricable and circular relationship between overt interpersonal interaction and intrapersonal processes that include unconscious fantasy and motive, object and self-representation, schemas, defenses, and cognition. As was noted in Chapter 2, these intrapsychic variables are believed to be maintained by ongoing patterns of relatedness in which other people are drawn in or are "hooked" into the roles of "neurotic accomplices" (Safran & Segal, 1990; Wachtel, 1993). The behavior of such partners in pathology serves both as a stimulus to and as a reinforcement of pathological behavior patterns and the internal processes that may either precede or be consequences of those interactions. Defenses or security operations (Sullivan, 1953) are seen as processes of avoidance that have a simultaneous intrapsychic and interactional impact in altering painful internal experience and in skewing new learning in social situations. The person cannot learn from experience and so is "stuck" in a perpetual state of re-creating and confirming his or her preexisting intrapsychic world at all levels of awareness (Andrews, 1993; Gold & Wachtel, 1993; Guidano, 1987; Safran & Segal, 1990; Wachtel, 1977, 1993).

In effect, integrationists who favor this perspective argue that the roles of antecedent and resultant, or of independent and dependent, variables are often interchangeable or, at least, are idiosyncratic and individualized. The outcome in terms of intervention strategies and tactics is a contextual, interactional expansion and elaboration of those used by the first group of integrationists. The major addition is the powerful underlining of the need to intervene actively in the patient's pathogenic interpersonal circles as they are manifested within current relationships, and in the therapeutic relationship. Integrative therapists of this persuasion therefore use such methods as assertiveness training, desensitization, cognitive restructuring, and contingency management to modify interpersonal patterns of avoidance, and to build new social skills that may eventuate in a lessening of fear and anxiety. In both cases, the theoretical assumption and clinical goals also include the point that these changes in conduct will test, clarify, and modify the associated modes of construing and representing experience at both conscious and nonconscious levels.

For example, as Wachtel (1977) pointed out, a patient's unconscious rage and sense of victimization at the hands of others, who are unconsciously perceived as powerful equivalents of persons from the patient's past, may be subjectively true if we examine the subtleties of the patient's current relationships. Her or his unconscious schemas, fantasies, and emotions are therefore more likely to change or to disappear following the establishment of more comfortable and egalitarian relationships than they might if insight were the single therapeutic goal. Also, active improvement in interactional abilities may lead to spontaneous insights in the form of newly recovered and symbolized memories, feelings, perceptions, and motives. Such intrapsychic material may then be met with further interpretive efforts and experiential exploration, or with additional active interventions.

All of these systems share a reliance on the strategy of tailoring behavioral, interpersonal, and cognitive interventions to best fit the patient's needs for change at those overt levels, at the levels of intrapsychic events, and at the level of the pathology maintaining interpersonal circles. Each individual system in this subgroup offers a strategic and tactical framework for active intervention that is structured by its unique theoretical integration. Wachtel (1977, 1993; Gold & Wachtel, 1993) has utilized the change mechanisms of exposure, gradualism, skills training, and contingency-based alteration of cognitive expectancies and behavioral consequences, all drawn from behavior theory and therapy, in combination with insight within an interpersonal and psychodynamic framework. His goals in changing overt behavior invariably include an understanding of the intrapsychic conflicts that shape and are reinforced by security operations in the interpersonal field. Standard behavioral interventions, instruction in communication and in interpersonal engagement, and more individualized techniques that combine dynamic and behavioral elements are considered with regard to the part of the circular process that dominates the clinical field. While behavioral measures are sometimes used in their most simple forms, they are usually designed within the perspective that accounts for the influence of symbolic and unconscious processes on new learning and its limitations.

In particular, Wachtel (1977, 1993) has been concerned with interrupting behaviors and interactions that are manifestations of disavowed and repressed anxiety, and that, if completed, reinforce and confirm the basic, unconscious patterns of defensiveness, avoidance, and encoding and construing the self and others. So, a technique such as assertiveness training is employed to help overcome a social skills deficit, which in turn may force the person to look at the unconscious sources of her or his social anxiety. Successes based on these new skills, in combination with these behaviorally derived insights, offer direct disconfirmation of the expectations and internal representations of the self and of others that were reinforced continually by previous social failures. This is just one example of the circular use of active work to promote multidirectional and many-leveled change in this system.

Guidano (1987), Horowitz (1988), Ryle (1990; Ryle & Low, 1993), and Safran (Safran & Segal, 1990; Reeve et al., 1993) have all developed contextually based integrative therapeutic systems wherein active behavioral, interpersonal, and cognitive exploration and exercises are used to promote changes in the patient's basic and deeply unconscious representational systems. Each of these authors has employed his own amalgam of structural cognitive theory with some version of a psychodynamically oriented interpersonal or object relations theory (see Chapter 2). They have concurred to a large degree that self- and object representations are embedded in and are reinforced and protected by overt patterns of interpersonal engagement, and further by conscious modes of perception and information processing. The tacit and nonconscious sphere of experience and the most overt levels of behavior are connected through certain mediating processes that are representational in nature and that serve automatic and redundant scripts (Horowitz, 1988), interpersonal schemas (Safran & Segal, 1990), or snags, traps, and dilemmas (Ryle, 1990). These mediational processes are conservative in nature in that they guide the person toward behavior that is familiar, secure, and avoidant of anxiety. Other persons in the patient's life are "hooked" (Safran & Segal, 1990) or induced into roles and behaviors that confirm the wisdom of such behavior, and that also reinforce the underlying schemas and representations. This last point is identical to Wachtel's (1977, 1993) notion of the vicious circle and of the role of neurotic accomplices.

Deep change, in the form of shifts and modifications in the internal personifications of the self and of others, as well as in the interpersonal schemas, tactical plans, and scripts, therefore requires change in the overt behavior and conscious modes of thought and perception that sustain and promote those tacit structures. These integrative clinicians rely on behavioral and cognitive exercises and experiments to induce such change. These active methods are placed firmly in the context of the interpersonal and relational patterns, guiding mediational plans and scripts, and overt expectations that require confrontation and disconfirmation. The patient is assisted through verbal and written exploration to being more aware of his or her thoughts, perceptions, schemas, and ways of "hooking" others. As such awareness unfolds, therapist and patient collaborate on the design, implementation, and evaluation of behavioral and interpersonal tasks. The unifying idea of such work is exposing patients to situations in which they must test their expectations of themselves and of others in ways and towards goals that they have avoided because of anxiety, conflict, or contradictory aspect of the self concept. Safran (Reeve et al., 1993; Safran & Segal, 1990) has relied on standard cognitive restructuring only when the patient is unaware of an irrational belief or dysfunctional thought, and therefore of its pathological effect. He has suggested that this approach is useful only infrequently, because the irrationality of most pathogenic thoughts is long known to the patient, to little avail. Safran has argued that such thoughts must be worked with in their interpersonal context. When they occur in the therapeutic relationship, the entire process of enactment or "hooking" must be identified, confronted, and tested, with the goal of both overt and covert change.

Ryle (1990; Ryle & Low, 1993) has used modified cognitive techniques, including extensive self-monitoring, log and record keeping, and cognitively based interpersonal exercises, as the central techniques of his cognitive-analytic therapy (CAT). These and selected behavioral measures are employed in the context of a structural and functional assessment of the person's self-and object representation, and of the ideational processes and behavioral sequences that reflect and confirm those unconscious structures. This assessment is offered to the patient in letter form. Written in everyday language, and emphasizing the overt attitudinal, behavioral, and interpersonal processes that express the underlying personality structure, this document becomes the key organizer of subsequent therapeutic activity. Maladaptive beliefs and disturbed interactions are selected for intervention on the basis of their role in confirming and reinforcing the representational structures and mediational strategies that are described in that letter. Additionally, the specifics of assignments are shaped to best meet the patient's need for an experience that will duplicate and then undo an inner object relationship or self-representation. For example, should the formulation include an inner relationship with a demanding and critical parent whom the patient feels must be placated, the therapy will focus on identifying and modifying interactions.

Confirmation of a maladaptive self-concept, through repetitive patterns of thinking, processing and representing experience, and engaging in relationships with others, is the central construct in Andrews's (1989) active self model of psychotherapy integration. He demonstrated a number of stages or levels of interaction within the self and with other people through which the basic processes of self-esteem and of identifying and characterizing the self may go well or go poorly. Essentially, this is a theory of the personally generated feedforward and feedback loops in which the self-concept is embedded. Like the other contextual models, Andrews's model views pathology as being derived from, and sustained by, the conservative and redundant interactions within the self, and with others, that serve the defensive purpose of avoiding anxiety and other discomforts at the cost of inhibiting any possibility of new learning or of modifying existing psychic structures.

Andrews (1993) suggested that active interventions are useful and appropriate at any stage of the process of self-confirmation at which the person is stuck. He advised the use of conventional behavioral, rational-emotive, cognitive, and systemic interventions as clinically indicated. Such methods are used with a dual purpose: first, of course, to produce the desired symptomatic changes, but more important, to disrupt the confirmatory processes that are implicated in the maintenance of a disordered or defective self. As active and didactic methods enable the person to behave differently, the feedback received by the self is altered, and the opportunity for new images, of, and attitudes about the self arises. These new opportunities occur both on an intrapsychic and an interpersonal level, depending where pathology has been corrected.

Westerman (1993) argued that behavioral interventions may be recast as one way the therapist can assist the patient to attain new, practical know-how, which in turn leads to the establishment of nondefensive and adaptive action patterns. In Westerman's hermeneutic model of psychotherapy integration, all effective intervention is thought to work toward that goal. The unique contribution of directed behavior change and education is the provision of direct examples of adaptive action patterns that serve as prototypes of other behavioral learning. In a similar vein, defensive interpersonal behavior may sometimes be abandoned or overcome by directed learning in such methods as assertiveness training, desensitization, or interpersonal skills training. When behavioral advances are made, the person becomes more aware of the sources of her or his anxiety and resistances to change. Such a pattern counters and undoes the self-maintaining and self-defeating circles of dysfunctional action and interpersonal relatedness in which the patient is trapped initially. Systemic techniques and strategic interventions (e.g., paradoxical intention) aimed at modifying repetitive interpersonal patterns are other types of directive intervention employed in this therapy. Again, the ultimate goal of such work is ending the maladaptive and self-reinforcing interactions that maintain the person's anxiety and pathology.

THE NARRATIVE APPROACH TO ACTION

The comedian George Carlin used to include in his stage act a routine about his behavior when he had found that he had lost his wallet. Carlin noted that, on discovering that the wallet was missing, he began to search for it. After looking in all of the typical and likely places and not finding it, he began a repetitive tour of his home. During this tour he would go back to the same spots again and again, only to find, "It's not back yet."

Psychopathology involves such a repetitive search for an answer, a solution, a prize, and like the comedian, the disturbed person makes the same choices, looks in the same places, thinks the same thoughts, and tells and confirms the same story again and again. This experiential and behavioral redundancy is a direct consequence of the dysfunctional life story that guides the person's adaptation. The disturbed narrative can often be changed best through direct changes in action. As the person lives differently, he or she may for the first time become aware of the critical part of the story that has caused life to be unfulfilling, frightening, or overly sad, lonely, or cruel. These discoveries may then lead to the evaluation of the inner attachment to such ways of construing and representing experience, with the potential for the development of fresh and more adaptive story lines about the self and others. Active work on these new themes and plots may then allow the person the rewarding experience of testing, refining, accepting, or letting go of new ideas, feelings, and interpersonal strategies, in the context of the safety of the therapeutic relationship. This experience also allows the incorporation of the therapist's responses to change, often countering or correcting forbidding, inhibiting narrative units that have been acquired in past relationships.

It may well be the new intrapsychic and interpersonal feedback that accrues from behavioral change that is the most important consequence of active intervention. There is no better way to establish a new story about oneself than to live it fully, in action and with deep access to the meaning and emotional impact of that story. As people respond differently to a change in behavior—say, greater assertiveness and self-confidence gained through behavior rehearsal and cognitive restructuring—they find much potential raw material to rewrite the themes and scripts that have not worked. The attainment of new behavioral skills that are based on changes in intrapsychic functioning, such as the ability to tolerate anxiety, that derive from learning to use soothing self-talk or calming imagery also evokes new and highly charged images of oneself as competent, intelligent, healthy, and so on. Finally, mastery over overt symptoms, such as being able to use air travel or to speak in public, offers the same opportunities for the revision of long-held narrative structures.

However, as was discussed earlier when we considered resistance (Chapter 4), people are often attached to their old patterns, problems, and ways of describing experience. We all know, professionally and personally, many people who are unable to attend to, to believe, or to assimilate the useful feedback that is offered by their own behavior and by the responses of others to them. An example of this type of narrative stickiness can be found in the literature on the "imposter syndrome." This label refers to the large number of competent and successful people who seem to be unable to trust and to believe the image of themselves that is accepted and reflected back to them by friends, colleagues, employers, and spouses. These persons deny, negate, invalidate, or ignore data that they could use to construct a narrative framework vastly different from and much more comfortable than the one that they tenaciously but often unwittingly protect and emphasize. The behavior of a well-known actress at an Academy Awards ceremony a number of years ago comes to mind in the context. When presented with the best actress award, she said to the audience, and perhaps a billion television viewers, "Now I know you really like me." This doubt about her acceptance by her peers and admirers had apparently persisted in spite of many choice movie roles, success in a couple of television series, critical acclaim, an earlier Academy Award, and great wealth. Her behavior speaks to how these data were not or could not be incorporated into her personal story. One wonders if the second Oscar was actually therapeutic in the long run.

The implications of this example are critical to understanding the broader role of, and the technical use of active interventions in changing, existing narratives. Cognitive and behavioral techniques are selected not only for their potential for internal and external changes in skills and adaptive patterns. While these changes are obviously valuable and important, by themselves they do not address optimally the crucial narrative structures and contents that lead to, and are reinforced by, these symptoms, excesses, or deficits. Consideration of the underlying narrational issue, and of the impact of the most salient piece of that issue, on more general functioning, guide the therapist in her or his choice of a technique. The therapist considers the potential for the generation of new experiences that will fill in a gap in the story, will correct the way the patient characterizes the self or others in response to herself or himself, or might highlight or push out of view some part of the story that needs more or less attention paid to it. Sometimes, cognitive and behavioral interventions can be used directly to this end; at other points, they may have to be modified or used in novel ways in order to meet the simultaneous goals of active change and narrative reconstruction.

As an example of the latter use, consider the patient whose fear of medical examinations had led to several situations that had placed his health in serious jeopardy. As this fear was explored, it seemed that it reflected themes of intrusion and vulnerability to authorities, as well as a sense of lack of control of his own body, both of which evoked powerful feelings of embarrassment and humiliation. The patient was an extremely intelligent man who held a doctorate in a scientific field and was extraordinarily well informed about biology and medicine. Therefore, I decided to work to expand his sense of power and authority, which existed and which worked well for him with his colleagues and competitors, to include his view of physicians. My assumption was that if he could demonstrate his competence to himself and to a physician before an examination, he could revise his view of the procedure to one in which he was respected and in greater control, and to one that was aimed at helping him, rather than humiliating him. We therefore worked up a plan for the patient to interview any number of physicians, to work at impressing them with his knowledge and skills, to explain his needs for control and respect during any exams, and to evaluate the reactions of these persons. We then worked on interview skills through the use of role playing and modeling, and we used some anxiety reduction techniques (relaxation, imagery, and self-talk) to ease his way into the process.

The patient interviewed a number of physicians, some of whom confirmed his ideas about their authoritarian lack of respect. In doing this, he began to separate these attitudes from himself, in that he was better able to recognize that these reactions meant more about physicians and their training than they did about him. He also dealt with a few individuals who seemed pleased by his efforts, who were interested in making him comfortable, and who offered the potential for a collaborative experience. This experience bolstered his view of himself as being safe and in control, and it enabled him to visit a doctor and to undergo a series of uncomfortable tests. This change led to a powerful and broad reworking of his old tale: He saw himself as having forever been unable to influence important people to attend to his needs, or to be sure of maintaining his self-respect when he was vulnerable.

In this case, as in most, the patient could not always use the feedback his new thoughts and actions generated. Perhaps the self-protective response to old, dysfunctional narratives is universal. At such times the therapist must focus carefully on the ways of, and reasons for, protecting the pathogenic story. This, focus requires detailed and sometimes prolonged inquiry into the details of the feedback to which the person was able or unable to attend; the ways in which he or she ignored, distorted, or avoided learning about the impact of the changes; and the emotional and psychodynamic reasons for these resistances. As a result, the narrational use of active intervention is frequently intertwined with an experiential and interpretive exploration of the impact of those interventions and changes on the person's experience of herself or himself and of others, and on the narrative frame that the therapist hopes to influence. This interweaving of the three domains of intervention is illustrated in the case example that continues in the next section.

CASE EXAMPLE: JAMES

In order to construct a new, healthy narrative, James needed to experience himself behaving in ways that contradicted the story with which he had come to therapy. Specifically, James had to observe and feel himself being successful in interactions with other people. He required the raw data out of which he could revise his portrayal of himself to include a self-concept that admitted the hope and possibility of being loved, and of finding happiness and satisfaction outside the narrow arena of work. His dealings with others also had to be changed to allow James to understand that people in his life could be benign, could be interested in his needs and well-being, and, on occasion at least, might be pleased and happy to know him at a more personal and intimate level.

The pathological life story that James had constructed had kept him insulated and isolated. As smart and as well informed as he was about most matters intellectual, he had done little learning in the social realm of life. He was awkward, uncomfortable, and unsure about the interpersonal acts that most people take for granted. In particular, he was filled with anxiety and had many obvious gaps in his thinking and behavior when called on to talk to his neighbors, relatives and colleagues when the subject was outside a work-related topic. In particular, James found it impossible to believe that anyone would want to know anything about him, his interests, his history, has feelings, or his goals. These behavioral and cognitive issues fed back into James's "machine" narrative and into his view of himself as a misfit and as one who stood outside the conventional social world. Therefore, as this narrative unfolded and was worked with interpretively and experientially, it was also necessary and important on many occasions to intervene behaviorally and cognitively. By the therapist's correcting his pathogenic beliefs and gradually helping James to fill in the gaps in his social learning, James was able to test his old narrative in the most immediate way. As, or more, important, James also accrued new interpersonal experiences that became another foundation for a more positive and healthy vision of himself in relation to others.

One of the first behavioral interventions, a technique that was used at many points during this therapy, was response cost. This intervention was suggested in order to move James out of the sealed world of work in which he lived, and into a wider range of experience. Response cost was also crucial in aiding him to face the enormous anxiety he felt about not doing a perfect job, or about leaving his office at a reasonable hour when an assignment had not yet been completed. These changes, which were discussed openly and were mutually decided on, were aimed at deeper levels as well: at showing James that he could survive the event of failing to live up to his perfect image of himself, that he could live differently from his workaholic father, and that he could tolerate and live through anxiety that had previously seemed unbearable.

The response cost was attached to the hour at which James left work. The cost of staying late was derived from the discussion of his relationships with his family. It became apparent that the idea of hurting his children was even more painful to James than was the anxiety that arose from leaving work unfinished. This cost was first identified through an interpretation of his repeating his relationship with his father in his dealings with his own children. As the sadness and pain became conscious, these emotions were expanded and deepened by means of a short series of experiential dialogues in which James talked to his now-grown children about his impact on their development. As he imagined the hurt and pain that his absences had inflicted, he became more determined to face his anxiety about work. We then decided that he would, on his own, remind himself of these dialogues and reopen them by himself whenever he was faced with a choice about leaving work on time or staying in order to reduce his anxiety.

Over a number of weeks, this intervention allowed James to get home at much more reasonable hours. He made several discoveries that were explored interpretively and experientially, and that set the stage for more behavioral change and narrative revision. First, he found that he enjoyed being home, that his wife was warmer and more sexually responsive, and that he enjoyed being with his children. Second, he found that his catastrophic levels of anxiety gradually lessened and did not predict any real catastrophes, and that his employers were merely mildly disgruntled. Last, he realized that he was stronger than he had believed, and that he could be a different person and could have a different life from his father's.

These changes in his view of himself took months to incorporate fully into his life story. As they were incorporated, he became more aware of the pain, isolation, shame, and anger with which he had unknowingly lived. As he became more hopeful of a different outcome to his narrative, James began tentatively to make overtures toward others in hopes of friendship. The awkwardness and uncertainty that had been his legacy often got in his way, and we became aware, from his reports and from the therapeutic interaction, of how his social skills deficits caused him to be hurt by others and thus reinforced his predictions of failure. Therefore, any number of sessions were devoted to discussions of social behavior, to role playing, assertiveness training, and behavior rehearsal. Also, the self-defeating cognitions that centered on his unlikability and his need to please others were explored and tested and became the impetus for homework assignments.

These behavioral interventions were interwoven with periods of dynamic exploration and experiential search. The act of learning from another man was fraught with meaning and emotion for James, as it exposed him to the significant lacks in his developmental history, and to the explanations and feelings that he had constructed to integrate and avoid the realization of his parents' distance and unavailability. At times, he would fail to remember or to complete exercises and would slip into his intellectual, argumentative mode when these omissions were pointed out. Interpretation of the underlying transference issues, and/or the active experiential enactment of the unfinished business with his parents, was often these impasses and to put into action the changes that had been suggested.

As he incorporated minimal, then moderate, and finally some major social successes, his deepest sense of himself as an asocial machine became conscious, as did an outpouring of grief and rage over what he had never had and had lost. As a result, these cognitive and behavioral gains several times precipitated therapeutic crises that required much dynamic, cognitive, and experiential exploration. It became apparent to both parties that James was now fully aware of the inaccuracies and the destructive impact of his existing narrative but felt imperiled by its loss. This story provided some sense of certainty, as well as familial continuity. These issues once again required a combination of insight, emotion, and active change: James had to put together a new awareness of the lack of surety and protection that accompanied a new and evolving narrative, to feel and to assimilate the separation from his family and the loss of his identification with it, and find the joy, power, and freedom he experienced in living out his new story.

III

Philosophical Concerns

8

The Worldview of an
Integrated Psychotherapy

This last chapter departs from a discussion of the theories and methods of psychotherapy and psychotherapy integration. Instead, it contains some thoughts about the worldview of psychology, psychotherapy in general, and the nature of theory and epistemology in the study of human beings.

THE MYTHOLOGY OF NATURAL SCIENCE OR A SCIENCE OF MYTHOLOGY?

The task of conceptualizing a fully integrated psychotherapy goes far beyond the important theoretical and technical considerations that have been addressed in the previous chapters. Critics of psychotherapy integration remain active and vociferous in their dire descriptions of the folly of work such as that represented in this book. Recently, for example, Lazarus (1995) repeated his well-reasoned and very persuasive argument that, while a technically eclectic psychotherapy is possible and desirable, theoretical integration cannot work successfully. This argument is based on Lazarus's refusal to accept the idea that the various theoretical systems of psychotherapy, particularly psychoanalytic theories, can coexist within a larger metatheory. In his view, the concepts contained in these theories are mutually exclusive and, in the case of psychoanalytic models, too far from empirical validation to be employed by a scientific, data-driven model

189

of treatment. Similarly, Fischer (1995) suggested that efforts at building theoretically integrated models of personality, psychopathology, and behavior change are based on certain erroneous myths about the component theories: that these theories are equally valid, can explain the same phenomena equally well, and therefore all deserve a place in future versions of therapeutic theory.

In my view, these arguments miss the point for a number of important reasons. First and foremost is the equation of theory and practice in psychotherapy with natural science and its methods of experimentation and theory building. Psychotherapy is *not* a natural science method, and its theories cannot be evaluated according to the same criteria as are theories in chemistry, physics, or astronomy. We work with and study human subjects and interactions between humans, who typically are not as mindless as chemicals, subatomic particles, or stars. The revolution against locating psychotherapy within a natural science framework has a long history, but it has blossomed since the mid-1970s with the rise of the narrative and constructivist psychologies that inform this book, as well as many others.

A constructivist discipline considers how its active subjects make sense and meaning of the raw data of their experience. This experience includes all of the subject matter of psychology and of the many competing sectarian schools of psychotherapy: wish, conflict, image, perception, ideation, emotion, behavior, and social action. The validity of such aspects of experience cannot and should not have to be proved or disproved. Rather, we hope to construct a theory that will allow each psychotherapeutic dyad to consider all aspects of experience in the most meaningful and pragmatic way possible. The narrative metatheory that is presented here is one attempt to create such a system.

Lazarus (1995) and Fischer (1995) represent a position within the natural science model of psychology that is to be explored in the next section of this chapter, on the distinction between process and outcome. The natural science model dictates a relationship to theory and method that in my view is just too inflexible and literal. To criticize integrative psychotherapists for their implicit myths is to fail to understand that all of our theories are nothing more than our shared, explicit mythologies (theologies, stories, narrative, and constructions). In fact, can we truly argue that the various psychotherapies actually exist and are practiced as they are described? Most of us are familiar with the nostrum that writings about psychotherapy are two steps removed from its practice: There is what we do, what we think privately about what we do, and what we tell others about we did. Here, then, is an example of the power of storytelling or myth making. In conversations with some of my more honest and secure colleagues, I have heard them state that they were influenced *after the fact* by what they had written about psychotherapy; that is, their ideas and methods had been shaped by the stories that they had told to themselves and others.

The methods of natural science *may* possibly be appropriate for evaluating psychotherapy, though to date all the research has yielded is a kind of equivalence of effect between systems (Luborsky, 1995). It is hubristic and incorrect to argue that some of our theories approach the truth about human existence while others do not. To the persons who created some of those theories, those insights and ideas were as compelling and useful personally as are the myths of natural science to the critics of psychotherapy integration. As Gill (1994) argued, the hermeneutic science of understanding how any individual creates and registers meaning can be validated not by prediction but by correspondence: Does the theory make useful sense of the process?

In concluding this chapter and book, I want to review two issues that in my mind bear directly on the arguments for and against the value of the pursuit of an integrated therapy. Attacks on theoretical integration seem to me to fit into the older and larger debate about process versus outcome in psychotherapy and psychology that have troubled this field throughout its history. This issue will receive further attention below, as will another. As I have worked through the years as a student and practitioner of psychotherapy, I have participated in what I now believe is one subset of the natural science ideology, namely, the silent but powerful idea that progress in psychotherapeutic theory and method comes from the therapist. I currently believe that we have ignored the contributions patients can make to our understanding of how and why therapy works and doesn't, and whether or not therapies can be integrated successfully. Below I describe how I have observed patients taking charge of their therapy and, in the process, creating what they (and I) experience as truly and profoundly integrated experiences. These events have highlighted the need to avoid the trap of the natural science model of observation, in which the observer's point of view is, to some degree, equated with "real data." We who write and think about psychotherapy have not often acknowledged that the therapist's point of view is taken as important without regard for the point of view of the other person involved in the process.

BRIDGING THE GAP BETWEEN PROCESS AND OUTCOME ORIENTATIONS IN PSYCHOTHERAPY

Psychotherapy has always existed somewhat near the fringe of mainstream academic psychology. This is especially true of those versions of psychotherapy that were generated elsewhere: in the offices of private practitioners, in medical centers, or in other relatively isolated settings. It is even more true of certain forms of psychological intervention that are built around a process orientation. That orientation, which is typical of psychoanalytically oriented psychotherapy, humanistic, experiential, and existential therapies, involves a relative disregard of the moment-to-moment visible signs of progress or improvement in the patient. Instead, these therapies share an investment in internal validity and in the signs of deepening and ever more broad immersion in the processes of self-understanding and experience.

Psychotherapy and academic psychology have at best coexisted uneasily throughout their respective histories. Scientific psychologists and clinical practitioners have condemned each other's concepts, ideologies, goals, and methods and have fought each other for the control of university departments, journal space, and professional organizations. At times, an uneasy rapprochement has appeared to emerge, and yet, the tensions between the two groups and their respective worldviews keep reappearing relatively unchanged. A key and central ideological and conceptual difference between the two positions, which has also translated into methodological conflict, has been the differing emphases on outcome measurement versus immersion in the subjective clinical process. Traditionally, scientists and practitioners have argued that one or the other is of utmost importance, while relegating outcome or process to the scrap heap if either is not dominant in the chosen framework.

This struggle also manifests itself within clinical psychology and psychotherapy as an ongoing dispute between those clinicians who identify with and seek to use the scientific methods and empirical findings generated by general academic psychology, and their opposites, who rely on psychodynamic, experiential, and humanistic theories and techniques that have never quite made it into the mainstream of psychological science. Scientifically aligned therapists have been known to scoff at the "softheadedness" of their counterparts, and to cite the untested and empirically vague status of the theories and methods espoused by the dynamic and humanistic groups. Correspondingly, this latter group has traditionally expressed its disdain for the scientific side of psychology by ignoring its principles, standards, and achievements, and by characterizing psychological science as superficial and relevant only to the simplest of clinical phenomena.

The original and ongoing causes of the estrangement between academic psychology and process-oriented psychotherapy are many and complex. They range from genuine and impassioned concern about the "truth" and about the development of psychological theory and method in the purest and most valid senses, to the more mundane and common issues of economics, prestige, and power that motivate and plague all professions and scientific disciplines. As Kuhn (1962) pointed out, only a small part of progress in research is aimed at, or accomplishes, the goal of learning something new. Much study in psychotherapy and in general psychology can be fit into this view of things.

Process- and outcome-oriented therapies and psychologies start and end with basic differences in understanding and working toward the alleviation of symptoms, suffering, and dysfunctional behavior.

A psychology that emphasizes the study of cause and effect, and that evaluates the utility of its independent variables in terms of an immediate, visible impact on clearly defined criteria, is the model of both research and clinical practice in an outcome orientation. Scientific psychology excels in the operational definition of its independent and dependent variables, and the therapies that have grown out of this tradition are marked by their insistence on clarity of concepts and by the need to specify behavioral referents for all constructs. Yet, scientific and outcome-oriented psychologies and therapies are often less effective when they are involved in the study and utilization of the intervening variables that are the "stuff" of process-oriented therapies. As a result, the former are construed by process theorists and practitioners as excessively empirical, empty, and superficial. Correspondingly, process approaches are criticized by more empirically focused psychologists as mentalistic; vague; dependent on loose, confusing, and redundant terms and concepts; and lacking any specificity with regard to the mechanisms and manifestations of change.

It is this gap in method and perspective that has kept these two camps apart, although I suggest that the integration of psychotherapies is one of the ways in which the gap has been and will continue to be breached. Standard versions of behavior therapy and cognitive therapy best exemplify clinical work based on an outcome model. The patient's symptoms and pathological patterns of action are the explicit targets of intervention. Progress in therapy is evaluated specifically in terms of the degree to which the targeted problems have been alleviated or modified. A process orientation proceeds from the premise that clinical change occurs indirectly, following from other, more ineffable, underlying changes in psychological and experiential structures, functions, and dynamics. This perspective is more closely related to the correlational methods of research, or to work in the arts, literature, or the humanities, where changes accrue in a somewhat unspecified or roundabout way following a reworking of basic foundations and principles of functioning. In fact, while a process therapy must be judged ultimately on its effectiveness in the reduction of psychopathology, its practitioners are advised to be "free of the desire to cure" (Freud, 1912) while the treatment is in progress. The process therapist shares with all healers a basic human concern for the plight of the patient and is, of course, motivated to help. However, the work of helping does not proceed in a straight line.

The major schools of psychotherapy that share an explicit process orientation, including psychoanalysis, the humanistic psychotherapies, the experiential and the existential psychotherapies, and interpersonal and systems therapies, also share certain clinical, conceptual, and epistemological assumptions and perspectives that are antithetical to a direct and emphatic focus on outcome and on measurable and replicable results.

Any psychotherapy that is conceived and conducted within a process orientation is based on a theory of personality change and of clinical intervention that is concerned with and selects inferred inner states and interpersonal cycles as the central issues to be assessed, understood, and resolved or changed. Overt behavioral changes are considered desirable but secondary and indirect by-products of effective and successful work on the experiential, affective, psychodynamic, or other intrapsychic processes identified in any specific process therapy. Change in the patient's functioning within the social environment and in her or his ability to adjust to reality demands is addressed infrequently, if at all, and again is thought to be the consequence of modifications in internal states and structures. In fact, certain varieties of process-oriented therapy are based on belief systems that argue against social adjustment and comfort as signs of health and of progress, viewing these variables as selling out to the norm (e.g., Fromm, 1955). For example, at various points since the mid-1970s, it has been argued that the typical personality that is "well adapted" to American society is the obsessive-compulsive, the narcissist, or the depressive. The Reagan years overvalued such character traits and drives as acquisitiveness, greed, and competition. Many process therapists would argue that successful therapy alienates an individual from a society that stresses and promotes such norms, rather than making the patient a "better citizen."

The methods and techniques of process-oriented therapies are almost exclusively verbal in nature. Interventions are used to move the therapeutic interchange away from conventional conversation to deeper aspects and spheres of psychological life, without a precise destination or end point in mind. An intervention is judged to be helpful or "correct" insofar as it affects the process of therapy by eliciting new material, by correcting an impasse or stalemate, or by enriching the patient's self-experience and self-awareness. Examples of such methods include existential confrontation, dynamic interpretation, and client-centered affective-reflective therapy. There are few if any external behavioral referents, goals, or outcome criteria attached to these clinical activities. The concepts that are used to describe and to understand the patient's verbalizations and the inferred covert variables that these reports represent have in the past been untested empirically and have been considered untestable by both the scientific and the process-oriented schools. For example, psychoanalytic interpretation is evaluated within a framework of internal validity. An interpretation is believed to have been helpful if it leads to process effects: the recovery of a repressed memory, a shift in the therapeutic alliance, or an integration of a previously warded-off image of the self, among others. The intervention is never judged directly with regard to its impact on the patient's presenting complaints. However, recent process work (see below) has been quite successful in applying to this type of data the rigor of definition and measurement that is part of outcome-oriented psychology.

Process therapies are traditionally evaluated by their practitioners and theorists on the basis of changes in the particular inferred intrapsychic states and variables that define each single system. For example, the client-centered therapist might look for greater congruence between the ideal self and the actual self, with a resulting expansion of awareness and symbolization of experience, while the psychoanalyst might assess therapy by using criteria such as enhanced insight and lessened repression of unconscious fantasy.

Behavioral change cannot be used as a criterion measure in most process-oriented therapies because of the uncertain and highly variable relationship between overt action and its presumed causative underlying processes. Many of these therapeutic systems include notions of over determination or of multiple causations of behavior that make the link between any single intrapsychic or interactional process and predictable behavioral change very loose or, in fact, impossible to construct. The emphasis in process models on symbolization, covert experience, and processes that mediate, alter, and distort consciousness and the expression of the intrapsychic in observable form also makes outcome a tricky and unreliable concept. Action is viewed as the final derivative of many possible intrapsychic events, interpersonal influences, and variables that are repressed, unsymbolized, or, in other ways—and for many possible reasons—unable to be brought into the individual's awareness. Therefore, the success or failure of process therapies cannot be scrutinized or conceptualized in a standard framework based on a directional model that assesses the impact of an independent variable on a specified behavioral criterion.

The ideologies and theories of many process-focused therapies clearly prohibit or disregard techniques and constructs that are aimed at overt changes in activity as final therapeutic aims and goals. Direct intervention in behavior is considered undesirable, useless, or even counterproductive in these therapies. Such direct intervention is construed as overly directive, reflective of the therapist's ideas or needs rather than those of the patient, and ultimately superficial and avoidant or obscuring of the more important and salient underlying processes and psychic structures.

The direction of psychotherapy by the therapist, in the form of overt, static treatment plans that target particular behaviors or experiences in an *a priori* fashion, also does not fit into a process orientation for theoretical and clinical reasons. The process-oriented psychotherapist operates from and within a stance of participation, exploration, and discovery vis-à-vis the patient. Therapeutic expertise and technical skill lie in the mode of facilitation of self-discovery for and with the patient. Successful work of this type requires attention to, and an ability for, the identification of and communication about subtle ripples and shades of intrapsychic and interpersonal experience. A prescriptive therapeutic stance that would result in outcome-oriented interventions requires the therapist to know in advance just which changes would be most beneficial for the patient, and how those changes can be promoted. This type and quantity of predictive and didactic knowledge is considered unavailable to the therapist in process models. Additionally, a prescriptive clinical stance is often seen as antithetical and detrimental to the therapist's capacity to assist in the patient's processes of exploration and expansion of awareness. The act of teaching or modifying the patient's behavior gets in the way of the discovery process, and it may cloud or impede that process in highly significant ways.

As should be apparent from the brief description above, a psychology that is dominated by experimentalism and reliance on observables cannot easily consider process-oriented theories and clinical methods. The conceptual bases and methods of the early forms of behavior modification, behavior therapy, and cognitive therapy grew out of, and were much more consistent with, contemporaneous trends in American academic psychology than were the psychodynamic, humanistic, or experiential psychotherapies.

Even in the present era, as psychology has been transformed by the cognitive revolution, the distance between process therapies and academic psychology remains severe and is to some degree increasing. As cognitive psychology and cognitive science have moved into the ascendancy in theory and research, the ever more specialized and sophisticated methods and concepts developed in those disciplines have not, with few exceptions (see, for example, the attempts to integrate cognitive and emotion theory with psychotherapeutic practice of Safran & Greenberg, 1991, and Stein & Young, 1992), been used to bridge the gap between science and practice. In a certain ironic fashion, new developments in outcome psychology have created process-oriented models that are consistent with the tools, constructs, and philosophies of outcome psychology. Cognitive psychology and cognitive neuroscience are increasingly concerned with how people build up working models of experience that operate outside awareness, and with how real experience and endogenous personality factors interact in the construction of these models (Stein & Young, 1992). Though the ideas, content, and implications of these new psychologies dovetail considerably with those of process therapies (for example, interest in mental representations and nonconscious functioning), the two groups remain significantly estranged. The reason is largely mutual unfamiliarity with the procedures, data, and premises of the other group, as well as the enduring and destructive rivalry and suspicion that typify relations between the lab and the clinic.

Process-oriented therapies will probably remain viable and vigorous, although in newly emerging, streamlined, briefer, and modified forms. Elsewhere (Gold, 1995), I have identified five areas of progress and change in process-oriented therapy. Each development represents a healthy and promising response to the challenges of outcome-oriented psychology or of the society at large to the standard theories and methods of process interventions. These advances include: (1) the development of empirically tested, manualized models of process therapy that are accountable in terms of outcome; (2) the simultaneous rise of short-term psychodynamic and experiential therapies that include an outcome-oriented, empirical focus; (3) research into the processes of therapy that have linked interactional and intrapsychic variables to change and improvement for the patient; (4) an increased interest in process concepts approaches among many members of the psychotherapeutic community; and (5) integrative theories and methods of psychotherapy that combine the process and outcome perspectives.

Each of these developments represents a unique and important integration of the strengths and contributions of the methods and concepts of both process and outcome psychologies and therapies. These integrations must allow for covert and overt processes to influence each other multidirectionally. They must also include both subjective and public vantage points in the evaluation process, with concern about internal and external changes. Finally, specified and replicable criteria for interventions, covert intervening variables, and outcome are necessary parts of these integrations. Each particular advance in process therapy can be seen to have addressed and included some, if not all, of these factors.

A discussion of all five of these advances is beyond the scope of this chapter (see Gold, 1995, for review). The main point I wish to make here is that the orienting role of integrative approaches allows psychotherapists to address process and outcome concerns within the same therapy. Narratives have outcomes that work and that don't, as they also have mediating processes between beginning and end that often deserve clinical attention. This theoretical approach makes many of the arguments between process and outcome approaches seem antiquated and irrelevant, particularly in light of the questions raised earlier in this chapter about the appropriateness of a natural science model for psychotherapy. By moving away from theories and methods that ignore the point of view of the subject (patient), we see that process and outcome are joined inevitably and inseparably. A constructivist theory, which frames clinical understanding and meaning in terms of the shaping of experience and behavior by an active individual, can be evaluated only in terms of the goodness of fit of the theory to the data, rather than through traditional modes of experimentation (Gill, 1994). As we have seen throughout this book, a model of integration based on narrative offers unique flexibility for therapist and patient to draw from the ideas and methods of both process and outcome traditions, and to avoid the ideological debates that have caused the schism between those approaches.

PATIENT-INITIATED INTEGRATION: TOWARD A FIRST-PERSON POINT OF VIEW FOR PSYCHOTHERAPY AND PSYCHOTHERAPY INTEGRATION

There may exist an important but untapped source of information that is germane to psychotherapy integration: the experiences, ideas, and actions of a certain subgroup of patients who have successfully integrated two or more forms of psychotherapy on their own. This group consists of patients who have been actively directed to or who have discovered ways to overcome their psychological and behavioral distress by conducting one of several forms of psychotherapy integration. These patients may be unique in that a significant number of them were psychotherapists themselves or were highly self-educated in the literature of the field. However, when approached somewhat conservatively, the self-reports and therapist observations of these persons may be highly enlightening. Reports of advances in psychotherapy integration share a common point of view with most articles in the field of psychotherapy. Clinicians or theorists write of their observations, interventions, and theoretical insights from the position of expert. In such writing, therapists are presented as the individuals who have made most, if not all, of the important technical decisions. Progress in treatment or in the elaboration of an integrative framework is typically described as a product of the therapist's intellectual and clinical efforts.

There are few clinicians who would argue with the necessity and value of this point of view. In fact, without such a mode of reporting, professional communication would be impossible. Yet, a significant source of bias is built into our writing and thinking. When we accept the subjective experiences of one member of a dyad (in this case, the therapist) as being preeminent, we often lose sight of the impact and value of the contributions of the other individual involved in the process (here, the patient). Such a discrepancy in evaluation may lead to clinicians' overvaluing their ideas and concepts and reifying what might better be considered tentative hypotheses, hunches, and metaphors. This bias may be of particular importance in the area of psychotherapy integration. Since this field is in its early days and is marked by debates over its feasibility, especially on theoretical grounds (e.g., Arkowitz & Messer, 1984), it seems critically important to broaden the data we use to evaluate and advance our work.

There are extremely few reports of patient-directed psychotherapy integration in the current literature (Bohart, 1995; Gold, 1994). Most schools of psychotherapy have moved to an egalitarian, collaborative position in which the patient's point of view is respected (e.g., Beck & Emory, 1985; Gill, 1982; Levenson, 1983; Reeve et al., 1993). However, the patient has not been described as the leader, innovator, decision maker, or creator of new forms of psychotherapy or of spontaneous integrations of psychotherapy.

Patients' perceptions of themselves and of the process of psychotherapy have been the focus of the second main area of research that is related to this topic. Perhaps the most significant source of this research is Frank's study of psychotherapy, *Persuasion and Healing* (1961), in which he identified the effective ingredient of psychotherapy as remoralization: assisting the patient to see himself or herself as capable and effective and instilling a sense of hope and optimism. This description is very consistent with the notion of self-efficacy highlighted by Prochaska and DiClemente (1992b) and has been expanded on by numerous other authors.

Shapiro and Morris (1978) argued that all gains in psychotherapy of any type can be traced to the modification of negative expectancies and to the development of positive perceptions of the self and the world, a position echoed identically by cognitive and rational-emotive therapists (Beck & Emory, 1985; Ellis, 1984). Strupp, Wallach, and Wogan (1964) were able to demonstrate that success in psychodynamic psychotherapy was predicted by patient perceptions of being liked and valued by their therapists and by similar positive perceptions of the therapist by the patient. Another study (Gold, 1980) followed up on the work of Strupp et al. (1964) by studying the expectations and perceptions of patients who were treated in behavior therapy. This study found similar relationships between the outcome and the perceptions of the therapeutic relationship.

Several studies of patient perceptions of the central and most efficacious events in psychotherapy highlight the potential discrepancies between an assessment made by a second party (the therapist) and by the patient. These findings impact on my ideas, which take as their starting point the notion of the patient as my active interpreter of his or her own needs and solutions. For example, it was found (Gold, 1980) that patients in behavior therapy saw the relationship with the therapist as equal to, or as exceeding, the specific therapeutic techniques in impact and importance. Llewelyn (1988) studied therapist and patient perceptions on a session-by-session basis. Both therapists and patients were asked to identify the most helpful events that had occurred in each session. Large discrepancies between the outlooks of the two groups were found, and these differences were most exaggerated in the small number of patients whose outcome was poorest. The patients noted understanding, relief, and reassurance as most important in their progress, while the therapists emphasized awareness and insight.

Glass and Arnkoff (1988) compared patients' perceptions of their own abilities to utilize certain behavioral and cognitive techniques with their stated preferences for such methods. Therapists' evaluations of the patients' abilities were gathered also. They observed that therapists' ratings of ability often did not coincide with the patients' ratings of their own skills, and that subjective self-evaluations frequently did not match stated preferences. These investigators also studied the explanations of therapeutic change offered by patients receiving one of four group therapies for shyness and social anxiety: social skills training, cognitive restructuring, problem-solving therapy, and unstructured group therapy (a control). The patients who had received the three active therapies attributed most of their progress to the individualized methods they had experienced, but there was also considerable mention of nonspecific relational factors, such as social support, feeling accepted and feeling understood. The group process was identified by the subjects in all conditions as a significant change-producing factor as well. Clearly, with the potential for such gaps in the construal of psychotherapy between patient and therapist, attentiveness to the patient's perceptions, plans, and hypotheses is critical.

The work of Shapiro (1981) and his colleagues at the Sheffield Psychotherapy Project actually combined investigations of combining different therapeutic approaches at different temporal points with an exploration of the subjective impact on the patients who had received such therapy. The investigators were able to tease out the relationship between treatment modality, patient perception, and type of change.

Llewelyn, Elliot, Shapiro, and Hardy (1988) studied depressed and anxious adults who had received eight sessions of both cognitive-behavioral and insight-oriented psychotherapy. They obtained self-reports from all subjects with regard to their perceptions of the most helpful and most hindering events in the two treatments. The experiences judged by patients to be most helpful were increased awareness, obtaining problem solutions, reassurance, and personal contact. Solutions to problems and reassurance were more likely to be gained during the cognitive-behavioral phase of therapy, while more expansion of awareness and personal contact were reported in the insight-oriented phase. The most troubling event reported by patients was the occurrence of unwanted negative thoughts, which occurred about equally in both phases and which were negatively correlated with outcome. Barkham, Shapiro, and Firth-Cozens (1989) looked at the same sample described in the Llewelyn et al. (1988) study to determine whether the order of the therapy phase (cognitive-behavioral followed by exploratory therapy or vice versa) affected the patients' perception of either phase of therapy or of the therapy as a whole. They found that the two phases had been experienced most differently by those patients who had received cognitive-behavioral interventions first.

This study was followed by another by Stiles, Barkham, Shapiro, and Firth-Cozens (1992), who found that the discontinuity produced by the initial phase of cognitive-behavioral intervention had been a product of the predominance of poorly formulated problems in the sample of patients. This type of problem was found to be most immediately amenable to the expanded awareness and personal contact that are typical of insight-oriented interventions. These gains lead more easily and effectively into a second phase of cognitive work. For a group of patients whose presenting problems were vague and uncertain, cognitive interventions were found to be more difficult and uncomfortable to assimilate initially.

In sum, the two areas of research just described argue for a perspective on psychotherapy that values and validates the patient's subjectivity and input, and the respects his or her need for different experiences, methods, and theories at different times. These findings dovetail considerably with the perspective presented here.

In these pages, I would like to raise these questions: What happens when and if the patient is in the driver's seat and the therapist goes along for the ride? Can psychotherapy integration benefit from the study of clinical and conceptual shifts that are initiated by the patient? Do our arguments and discussions about eclecticism or integration (Lazarus, 1992, 1995), seamless integration (Wachtel, 1991), visions of reality (Messer & Winokur, 1984), or levels of integration (Schacht, 1984) change or grow when we consider the patient's role as an active participant in the integrative process?

What follows are observations of four ways in which patients have taken the lead in the clinical situation and have changed an on going therapy into a truly creative and integrative experience. Each mode of integration employed by the patient was utilized by that individual out of a sense of reaching his or her personal goals for a healthy, comfortable, and satisfying life. The novel and individualized therapeutic experiences initiated and created by these patients appeared to be integrative in the truest sense of the word. These persons described their choices as fitting into and comprising some useful sort of gestalt.

These patients reported that the different interventions and theories were intrinsically linked and were necessary if they were to achieve the best results by their own standards of evaluation. The disparate therapies were synergistic and not at all contradictory at an ideological or experiential level. These integrating patients perceived dynamic, cognitive, behavioral, and humanistic methods and ideas as intrinsically interconnected in a nonlinear way. In addition, as a group, they seemed to agree that thinking about these different levels of experience, and subsequently choosing to work therapeutically in several or all of those areas, was most advantageous if not absolutely necessary. Because of these reports, it seems valid and appropriate to discuss these cases as modes of integration that are considered, chosen, and completed by the patient, rather than as haphazard or syncretistic forms of therapy.

Mode 1: The Integration of a Sequence of Therapies

Mode 1 is probably the most common way in which patients in psychotherapy manage their own treatment. It involves selectively seeking out one form of psychotherapy of a specific type and on completing work in that modality, seeking out another form of therapy for deliberate reasons. In this mode of integration, the patient takes an overarching view of his or her life plans, psychopathology, ambitions, needs, and wishes and constructs a "grand psychotherapy" that is composed of two or more parts. This approach to and participation in psychotherapy is not an aimless form of searching for answers. Exploration of the therapeutic choices made by these patients reveals that they may have a viable and unified vision of what they want, need, and in fact know would best alleviate their personal difficulties and assist their movement toward health. This sense of potential growth guides their choices and leads to an integrated experience of psychotherapeutic involvement. This experience is salient and stable even though the therapy is carried out in stages and with different therapists and modalities of therapy. Here, we find true integration at the experiential and phenomenological levels of living.

The patient who embarks on a sequence of differing psychotherapies usually does so by educating herself or himself about the types,
benefits, goals, and disadvantages of several methods of psychotherapy. Once this information has been assimilated, a process of consideration and matching seems to occur. Patients report that decisions
to undertake a second, third, fourth, or more rounds of treatment are
influenced by conscious and unconscious factors that grow out of
particular concerns. Most important, the patient sifts through the
positive changes accrued in initial therapies, looks at his or her unfinished issues, and synthesizes these perceptions against the backdrop of the stored information about alternate therapeutic choices.
The person's final decision is influenced by the felt need to address
and to expand experiences that were limited in a previous therapy,
by the need to expand earlier gains through work in different areas
of experience, and by an awareness of assets and potentials that were
not tapped by the previous treatment.

Persons who construct an integrated sequence of psychotherapies
are unlike those patients who seem to be "shopping" for therapy in
a casual and nonserious way. The latter group appears to be engaged
in some conflicted or compromised activity aimed as much at avoiding
therapeutic involvement as at obtaining it. The active management of
a therapeutic sequence implies a powerful orientation toward the future. The integrating patient may be unique in his or her vision of a
new, healthy identity and way of life, and in making an informed
plan of actualizing that vision. These variables may be missed by
therapists at any point in the sequence, particularly if a therapist is
made insecure by the patient's choices, or if a therapist has ideological
reasons for discounting the validity of the patient's integration and
management of his or her own care. However, careful and respectful
inquiry into these choices and their rationale often reveals the intelligent, thoughtful, and holistic decision making described above.

Mode 2: Concurrent Integration of Two Separate Therapies

Mode 2 of integration is a process in which a patient makes simultaneously use of two forms of psychotherapy. This decision is
usually prompted by the patient's sense of being stuck at a critical
point in one form of treatment, and of being unable to move past
that therapeutic impasse within the context of the first therapy. This
experience leads to a search for other theories and techniques that
will synergize with the work of the first therapy by providing new
and additional skills, experiences, or perspectives. As a result of such

additive integration, the patient maps out and follows a plan of therapeutic work that is consistent with her or his goals.

The typical path within this mode begins with a successful, ongoing experience in one type of therapy that runs into some kind of
protracted obstacle. The most frequent of such roadblocks is a symptom or personality trait that will not remit despite intensive efforts
by both parties. Such obstacles often become massive and unwork-
able, leading to hopelessness, despair, and an undoing of previous
therapeutic progress. All major systems of psychotherapy have explanations for such roadblocks, as well as suggestions for their management and resolution. In the situation described here, such approaches
have failed or have been circumvented by the patient's active decision
to overcome a roadblock through the addition of another therapeutic
approach. Usually, once the desired symptomatic or personality
change is made, the patient suspends involvement with the second
therapist. On many occasions, the skills and experiences that were
part of that second treatment are brought into the ongoing therapy,
should new roadblocks emerge. Some patients also will consult the
second therapist for repeated stints, or they add a different type of
therapy at a later point for another round of concurrent integration.

Patient-initiated choices of concurrent therapies are experienced
by the patient in much the same way as Mode 1 integrations. Both
therapies are seen as integral and necessary pieces of a greater therapeutic whole, and the methods and ideas of each component are construed as synergistic and complementary. The patient is guided by
his or her own needs, is free of the ideological and methodological
attachments that may inhibit a therapist, and therefore is sometimes
more free to create a new, "grand therapy" from two or more concurrent parts.

A critical piece of successful concurrent integration seems to be
respect for the patient's choices, and for the work of each therapist's
counterpart. It would be easy and natural for the first therapist to
construe the choice of a second ongoing treatment as a statement of
hostility, resistance, triangulation, or other such important conflicts.
Such a perception is sometimes valid and correct. However, at other
times, particularly when a well-conducted therapy has bogged down
and cannot be unstuck conventionally, the decision to add another
modality may be an expression of the healthiest and most creative
striving in the patient. If, for personal or theoretical reasons, the therapist cannot recognize the possible validity of concurrent integration,
the patient may abandon the idea or engage in a second therapy in
a way that compromises both parts of the integrated therapy. Simi-

larly, the second therapist may welcome the patient's choice out of a sense of vindication, competitiveness, or pleasure at the failure of another therapist and therapy. If doing so, the necessary work in both aspects of the therapies may be endangered.

It is not uncommon for a psychotherapy patient to seek out two or more forms of help while continuing with the first modality. This most is frequently the case of those patients who decide to enter group therapy, couples therapy or family therapy, while continuing with their initial individual therapy. Also common is the decision by the patient to combine pharmacotherapy with an existing psychotherapy, or vice versa. However, the decision to combine two concurrent forms of individual therapy is rarely, if ever, discussed in the psychotherapeutic literature. This lack of attention may simply reflect the relative rarity of such a choice by patients. However, it may also reflect some of the negative reactions by therapists to such suggestions or decisions when arrived at by patients. This type of counter-resistance to integration initiated by patients is discussed in more detail below.

Mode 3: The Integration of Self-Therapy with Ongoing Therapy

Mode 3 of patient-initiated integration involves a search by the person for new therapeutic skills, techniques, and experiences that he or she can learn and apply without the formal assistance of a second psychotherapist. This process may commence as a response to some new learning experience in an ongoing psychotherapy. Equally commonly, such behavior is a response to the type of therapeutic stalemate that prompts Mode 2 integrations. In either situation, the patient becomes aware of some therapeutic work that he or she wishes to undertake or to complete and then seeks out the knowledge and methods that are necessary. This self-therapy is formulated and learned through reading, tapes, lectures, or other popular and professional materials. Once the person feels that a sufficient level of competence has been reached, that individual begins to treat himself or herself. The educational search, its cognitive and affective underpinnings, and the materials found sometimes become the focus of work in an ongoing therapy.

However, in certain cases, the therapist learns of the patient's self-therapy only *after* the patient has successfully completed a piece of self-therapy. One wonders about the numbers of patients who have conducted this form of integration and have never informed their therapists. This last point is interesting and important, particularly because it hints once again at the crucial role played by the therapist's conscious and unconscious attitudes toward the patient's leadership, control, and therapeutic vision and acumen.

It is likely that some therapists communicate their discomfort to patients who have used self-therapy modes of integration, thereby sabotaging the process and making the patient less willing to report on these activities.

Discussions with patients who have learned and applied alternate therapeutic methods and ideas while in an ongoing psychotherapy indicate that such persons experience their self-treatment as a holistic extension of their psychotherapy. Rarely do they believe that the self-therapy was more powerful than the formal psychotherapy. Most indicate that the ongoing psychotherapy freed them to use the alternate methods, and that the self-therapy potentiated the ongoing psychotherapy. Often, self-therapy was an effective way of coping with or resolving a stubborn symptom or behavior pattern that had become a major interference in the ongoing psychotherapy.

These individuals were also informative and enlightening with regard to their reactions to the theoretical and practical issues posed by learning about one school of therapy while being involved in another. Several patients indicated that they thought that their therapists took their own theories and ideas too seriously, and there was also a general consensus that these methods and foci were compatible and complementary. As noted above, these patients also stressed the therapist's interest in, acceptance of, and encouragement of self-integration as a major variable in the success of such endeavors.

Mode 4: In-Session Integrations of Interventions

Mode 4 of integration occurs when a patient uses a moment of therapeutic activity or experience as a springboard for work with alternative perspectives. Unlike the first three modes, it is more immediate, spontaneous, and unstudied, depending on a subjective sense of wanting to broaden or deepen the therapy. Those patients who have a professional or educational familiarity with psychotherapeutic methods may, of course, draw on that knowledge in these instances. But, it is most fascinating to observe patients reinventing and discovering psychodynamic, experiential, or cognitive-behavioral techniques, guided predominantly by the need to overcome a momentary therapeutic stalemate or by a wish to expand a piece of progress.

These integrations are of several related types. The patient may follow a dynamic insight or experiential change as a stimulus for developing a behavioral technique for modifying a troubling cognition. Such integrations express, implicitly or overtly, a need felt by the patient to "do something practical with what I've felt or realized." That is, insight begets a desire for action. Similarly, cognitive and behavioral change may be the impetus for dynamic work that leads to new insights or to the creation of an experiential exercise aimed at a deepened access to inner states. Here, the quest may be for "something I can do to get deeper into this and to see what's behind it." Thus, action stimulates a wish for insight.

Moments of feeling stuck or blocked while working in any of many modalities may yield a request or decision by the patient to shift perspectives. This change sometimes results in the invention of a new method, based on a different level or type of construal by both parties.

Sometimes, this mode of integration is completed only partially by the patient. In these instances, the patient is aware of a desire to change sets and methods but cannot come up with a specific intervention or with a previously learned technique. Instead, he or she requests such work on the therapist's part or may attempt to engage the therapist in a collaborative process of education or mutual invention.

Mode 4 makes particular demands on the therapist for a number of reasons, chief among them its immediacy in the session. Therapists are often trained to see unexpected shifts away from the work at hand as resistance, countercontrol, inauthenticity, or some other manifestation of pathology. At times, this mode of integration, like the others, may be employed by the patient to avoid anxiety, to obfuscate, to resist, or to express some interpersonal struggle in the therapeutic relationship. The optimal attitude on the part of therapist is openness, curiosity, respect, and a willingness to explore the potential validity of the patient's expertise in designing a personalized grand therapy. Such reactions are most likely to enable the therapist to identify those instances of patient-initiated integration that will promote progress and those that will prove counterproductive.

THE IMPLICATIONS OF PATIENT-INITIATED INTEGRATION

Integration initiated by the patient places unique and difficult demands on the psychotherapist. Cherished theories and techniques may be challenged by the patient in word or deed. The role and prescribed activities of a therapist in such a patient-controlled situation are unclear and lack the safety and familiarity that most of us welcome in our work. Clinical lore, psychotherapy theories, and empirical research are of little use in orienting the therapist's thinking or behavior. He or she may thus be forced into a seat-of-the-pants idiosyncratic response. The therapist must master two interrelated challenges simultaneously. One is a task of clinical assessment; the other is a process of self-exploration and understanding. Central to the therapist's clinical exploration of the patient's integrations is the need to determine whether these integrations represent some sort of positive and helpful process or a disjunctive and destructive phenomenona. Such conclusions on the therapist's part are highly vulnerable to the effects of his or her own construal of and emotional reaction to the patient's efforts, as well as to the therapist's allegiances to particular theories.

The patient may attempt to take control of the therapy for reasons, other than progressive ones, of which he or she may or may not be aware. We may place such actions in the category of resistance or countercontrol. But other causes of resistive interest in patient-initiated integration are the following. Patient-initiated integration may arise from the patient's need to avoid anxiety or other unpleasant inner states; from anger at, competition with, envy of, or hate for the therapist, in response to a rupture of the therapeutic alliance (Reeve et al., 1993); or from a need to sabotage the treatment. However, as the discussion of the four modes above indicates, this is not always the case. In my experience, the patient's integrative efforts are seldom a manifestation of resistance or of destructive tendencies.

There is no way to make an assessment of the meaning of the patient's integrations in an *a priori* fashion. Traditional theories may lead to a bias toward construing the patient's novel efforts as "not following the rules." But these same theories offer little guidance for understanding or identifying the covert or nascent stirrings of health and creativity in the patient. Therefore, it behooves the therapist to undertake a most careful and neutral exploration of the ideas, motives, feelings, and fantasies, that are stimuli to patient integrations. The therapist must examine the therapeutic relationship with subtlety to rule in or out unacknowledged alliance ruptures or transferential issues that must be corrected. The timing of the patient's integration and the status of therapeutic work just prior to the introduction of interest in integration may yield crucial information. It may be helpful to inquire of the patient whether his or her current integrative ideas are part of a large grand plan for therapy. If so, his or her integrations are placed in a different context from integrations that seem to have no foundation in the patient's beliefs or knowledge base.

Even if occasionally the patient's integrations are found to be a vehicle for resistance or some relationship problem, they require a respectful response from the therapist. Sometimes, the patient will give up an interest in a change in modality when the underlying issues are resolved. At other times, the patient will continue to believe in the wisdom and efficacy of such changes after that resolution. In those cases, it may be advantageous for the therapist to encourage the patient to go forward.

Optimal clinical exploration will be hindered to the extent that the therapist feels undermined, wounded, competitive, or in any other way hurt by the patient's efforts. Issues of grandiosity, helplessness, power, control, prestige, and authority are all germane to this discussion. The therapist who is invested in being the expert or the healer may be unable to identify the health in a patient-initiated integration. Therapists whose "guild" loyalties cause them to put down other theories and approaches will be at a disadvantage. Similarly, those clinicians who disrespect intellectual approaches to psychological problems, and who believe that educating oneself is an avoidance, will not be receptive. Therapists' exclusive ownership of knowledge and competence with psychotherapeutic methods are challenged severely by patient integrations. Also, "ownership" of the patient is attacked, in all of its economic, professional, and personal meanings, by the autonomous actions of the patient. This last point is most apparent in Modes 1 and 2, in which two therapists are hired by the patient to assist in her or his grand psychotherapy.

A final methodological point grows out of these observations. About a third of the patients who have successfully managed the integration of their therapy were therapists themselves. Most of the other patients were well educated and knowledgeable about psychotherapy. Those who lacked such education at the beginning of psychotherapy were resourceful enough to fill in the gaps in their education and experience with comparative easy. Perhaps, if therapists made information about the varieties of psychotherapy available to all patients at the beginning of treatment, more patients would be encouraged to be integrators.

Additionally, it may be appropriate to work with therapeutic stalemates and resistances by enlisting the patient in the design of therapeutic solutions and alternatives. This approach would also require making educational materials available and working with patients in more didactic and instructional ways. Therapists of many persuasions have endorsed such collaboration, education, and role induction.

The ongoing arguments about the validity and possibility of psychotherapy integration have invoked such variables as theoretical voice and vision (e.g., Messer, 1992) and theoretical compatibility (Franks, 1984; Niemeyer, 1993; Schacht, 1984). Discussions of this type appear to be based on an implicit acceptance of a natural science model of observation, hypothesis testing, and model building. Natural science models are built on a *third-person point of view* of description and understanding. Third-person theory building is all that is possible and necessary when the subject under study is inanimate or is unable to communicate with the observer. However, patients are sentient, communicative, and deeply concerned in their own experience. In particular, as has been stressed throughout this book, patients, like all of us, are capable of knowing their own stories and of being able to figure out how those stories should best be changed.

If, as Sullivan (1953) so brilliantly argued, personality is the trajectory of one's experience into the future, why would we as therapists choose to ignore the person's own view of that path?

"Third-person" psychotherapy theories do not invite or utilize the input of the subject under study. From the third-person point of view, we impute a story to a character, or we tell it about that person. We do not invite the telling of, reflection on, or active revision of the narrative by its own author. As a consequence, our theories tend to be experience-distant, reductionist, and incapable of capturing the nuances of the phenomenology of human life. Because each theory focuses on its part of the elephant, the differences between theories are be exaggerated. Hence, the debates and concerns about the appropriateness of theoretical integrations are exaggerated as well. And yet, when the consumers of these theories employ them, their experiential sense tells them (and us) that they overlap considerably, that they are frequently synergistic, and that they rarely act in opposition to each other. Perhaps the reason is that patients' narratives empower them to find overlaps where our ways of constructing experience have taught us just the opposite.

Some of the patients who have found their own integrative paths created personal theories that came to resemble existing integrative models. Other patients felt, on reading the psychotherapy integration literature, that certain writings best fit their experiences. Some patients appreciated and resonated to such systems as cyclical psychodynamics (Wachtel, 1993) and the active self model (Andrews,

1993). These writings often elicited comments on the order of, "If I were a psychotherapist, I would have written that," or, "That puts into words what I felt about myself." However, we rarely, at least in public, check out our methods and theories with our collaborators in therapy: our patients. Perhaps in failing to do so, we lose a major resource. Without theories that embrace patient-initiated integrations and include a first-person point of view, we may be stuck in taking third-person-dominated models too seriously and thereby blind ourselves to what our patients have to teach us about psychotherapy integration.

THE "INSIDE-OUT" PSYCHOTHERAPIST

To conclude this chapter and book, I would like to reflect on why integrative methods seem to "work" with some patients and not with others. In the therapy of some patients, the moves from voice to voice and from technique to technique that are described in this book seem natural, easy, and an organic part of the experience. Usually, at the time, and in retrospect, these shifts seem to be "right" in that they lead to results that are desired by both parties. Other therapies do not move, and changes in method and perspective are felt to be mechanical, wooden, and unproductive. For example, how would we explain the following event in a therapy session?

A patient recalls a positive exchange in his past therapy with another therapist moments after describing his frustration and lack of assertiveness in reaction to his mother's possessiveness and jealousy. He furtively looks at me and then away, smiles uncomfortably, and then begins to talk about current difficulties with his supervisor, who the patient feels is psychologically unstable and prone to verbal outbursts. Where, if at all, do I intervene? There are markers here that therapists of any stripe would recognize: experiential, cognitive, behavioral, and psychodynamic. As he talks, I recall Jehovah's Biblical injunction to the ancient Israelites to "have no other gods before me."

Am I the jealous authority? Or is it only mother, or the supervisor? The patient's discomfort in talking well of his previous therapist in front of me suggests that I am involved here. Is his discomfort conscious or unconscious and, if unconscious, to what degree? Are there affects that are unsymbolized, assertive behaviors to be shaped, dysfunctional cognitions to be examined? Is it any wonder that most of us would, at such a moment, feel great despair in choosing an option or would flee to the relative certainty of one of the established schools of therapy? At least that choice of a single theory would rule out most of these questions.

In the spirit of the narrative approach, I feel I might start to answer these question by telling two stories that seem very pertinent.

When I was a teenager, I spent much time playing rock music in a band. Along with disturbing the neighbors and ruining my eardrums, this activity was a source of great happiness even though, most of the time, the music never improved beyond the very mediocre. However, on certain occasions, something extraordinary would happen. Without planning or discussion, a jam session would evolve around the basic structure of a very familiar song or chord progression.

During these jams, the band would play extended improvisations that included solos for each member, as well as improvised ensemble work that would feature two or three of the lead instruments (guitars, piano, organ) playing melodically while the rhythm section of bass and drums supported them.

Each of the players seemed to know and to be able to anticipate the direction that his band mates were taking, without signal or discussion. The music that was made moved from tempo to tempo, rhythm to rhythm, and melody to melody without words, plan, or goal. Keys would change, solos would begin and end, all of a piece. Somehow, the individuals who made up the band sensed these rare moments in which the collective experience guided, shaped, and formed the music.

Musicians describe this experience as being in a "groove," or as finding the "lost chord." Athletes often speak of being "unconscious" and finding the "zone" that allows them to pass a basketball to a teammate without looking in her or his direction, or to anticipate the flow of a play on the field before it unfolds. Longtime friends and mates can often complete each other's sentences and find themselves simultaneously thinking of the same thing in a variety of circumstances.

In narrative terms, it seemed as if each band member had penetrated to the inner structure of the music, and in finding this unspoken architecture, something ephemeral and powerful was created: a collective work of art that could not have been written out or planned ahead of time.

The second story involves the question that I am asked in every course in psychotherapy that I teach. What my students want to know more than anything else is, of course: How does psychotherapy work? I tell these classes that I feel close to and comfortable with about a cartoon from the *New Yorker* magazine. In the cartoon, a blackboard fills most of the space, at the top of which is the heading, "The Physics of Creation," followed by a complicated mathematical equation. The equation ends with an asterisk, and at the bottom of the blackboard appears the footnote, "And then a miracle occurs."

I hope that I am not being too obscure here. The "miracle" that occurs in psychotherapy often seems to me to be the one that allows a bass player and a drummer to change tempos at the same time that the guitarist across the room moves out of his solo. We have in our theories of psychotherapy many terms that only partially capture the miraculous, collective experience that completes the therapeutic equation. These include *empathy, attunement, merger, collaboration, alliance,* and *transference and countertransference.* But these ideas merely describe and don't explain the miraculous ways that therapists make useful choices when faced with experiences as complex as the one I have spelled out in these pages. These terms all reflect what Cushman (1995) defined as the glorification of the bounded, individual self in American psychotherapy, as well as the scientism that we as a discipline aspire to attain. Western culture and science do not do a good job of learning and teaching about events in which two (or more) people may fuse their narratives. Other cultures that do not define the self as totally separate from others in the community are more inclusive of the notion of shared experiences and do not relegate these ideas to the fringe of thinking (i.e., do not dismiss these notions as "spiritual," "New Age," or "ESP").

Even Freud (1912) was aware of such phenomena, as he noted that the best interpretations in psychoanalytic treatment are those that result when the unconscious of the patient speaks directly to, and is recognized by, the unconscious of the analyst. Yet, we don't allow much room for discussions of how to get in the "zone," or about how to get the patient and the therapist to create a jam around some stale riffs, chords, and lyrics that both have heard before. In our zeal to be scientific, to test, replicate, and prove what we know, we may sterilize our observations and miss what is most important.

To conclude, then: The miracle of successful psychotherapy occurs when patient and therapist meld their minds and their experiences. A blurring of boundaries and of selves seems to occur, so that the patient's narrative gets woven around and into the experience of the therapist. Somehow, the healthy core of what could be and what might have been that is contained in that story comes to be known by both people, even if it cannot be discussed or articulated yet. This shared experience then may be the best guide to selecting the vision, sphere of psychological life, and type of therapeutic intervention.

When this interpenetration of lives and stories happens, the "next moves" in the relationship unfold as smoothly as Magic Johnson's behind-the-back pass to an unseen teammate, or as seamlessly as the Modern Jazz Quartet's collective decision to move from the key of A minor to the key of B-flat-minor at the thirty-seventh bar of a piece. When patient and therapist fail in this kind of connection, the therapy may be technically successful, but at a level that misses the organic wholeness of the most emotionally evocative therapies. How to accomplish such a melding of two persons is, of course, the final *Jeopardy* question.

I am far from the answer. I believe that these experiences result from a mutual desire, affection, courage, and curiosity and, on the part of the therapist, a willingness to suspend self-interest, and to taste and to experience from within, the life and experience of another firsthand. Probably, and this is a heretical statement from a psychologist-psychotherapist-academician, this type of encounter requires a belief in magic.

The Lovin' Spoonful asked if we believed in magic in a song from the late 1960s. Our literature, theater, music, and movies (all of our main cultural narrative sources) are filled with a longing for, and a terror of, magic. Teenagers (and many adults) fill their hours by playing magical, mystical video games and role-playing games. Yet, psychotherapy does not make much use of magic. We don't really acknowledge its place in our stories, because it is "primitive," "unscientific," and impossible to measure. But we can't make it go away. This phobic reaction to magic is unique to Western societies. In cultures that have retained more of a sense of the communal, magic as a metaphor for the transpersonal and the shared is given more credence and authority. We need only to look at the literature of eastern Europe (e.g., Isaac Bashevis Singer) or South America in the works of Isobel Allende, Jorge Luis Borges, or Gabriel García Marquez for examples of this power.

Stories are magical in their power to be politically subversive, to influence, to create new worlds, and to allow the teller of tales and the reader (listener) to escape from the constraints of reality for a while. Amos Oz (1995), the Israeli novelist and critic, argued that the storyteller receives, carries, and transforms the ghosts, goblins, and psychic terrors of the tribe through the sorcery of ordering and naming; giving voice and structure to what is known but not faced tames it. Winnicott (1971) suggested that effective psychoanalysis is made up of experiences that are playful and that escape the limits of reality. As noted earlier, Mitchell (1993) stated that freedom from psychopathology often depends on one's imagination. Bateson (1994) pointed out that the failure to learn from experience can often be traced to the existence of narratives that prescribe rigid constructions of reality, and that dictate absolutist worldviews. As a results, people and cultures are alienated from each other and from experience.

When the therapist can turn herself or himself inside out and can step outside the boundaries of the received notion of reality that tells us that we are monadic entities whose experiences stop at the limits of our skin, then perhaps magic can occur.

Magic, of course, is another metaphor or story about life. A belief in magic results from the need to explain and to control the unknowable and the awesome. Other stories may suffice for other therapists. About this, I have no complaint or argument, only that, if they substitute *scientific theories* for *magic*, they will realize that those theories are stories as well, chosen as much for their personal fit with the therapist's history and individual narrative as for their objectivity and truth. The philosophy of science is full of documentation of the large gap between empiricism and "truth" (Cushman, 1995; Kuhn, 1962).

Making magic, allowing ourselves to step outside our ordinary and conventional stories and ways of making sense of things, and to believe in magic, requires a world that has been disappearing for a very long time. The freedom to work slowly, a growing rarity these days, helps immensely, as does a therapist's freedom from anxiety and other pain, at least while he or she is in the session. The ability to play, and to suspend our attachment to being certain, to being right and, to our claims to expertise and authority may also be crucial. To allow the patient to express her or his narrative in the first person, and to enter into that narrative as a supporting player, is much more obscure and difficult for any therapist than to apply a third-person, objective construction.

Probably, we all draw on whatever rare form of communal, collective experiences we have had in our lives (as I did in referring to my brief musical involvement) to create stories and metaphors that seem to capture this kind of connection. My grandfather, Natan Sarotzkin, to whom this book is dedicated, made magic for me when I was young. A man who came from a world that was destroyed many years ago, both physically and socially, he told me the stories of his life, of the Bible, of people and places that I had never seen and would never see. In doing this, he shaped me, for better or worse, to be who I am, to belong to a community that exists in memory, tales, books, and artifacts, as well as in new places that he did not know himself when he was young. When my work with a patient goes well, and when somehow I find myself in the same key or on the same page with that person, I often feel Natan's presence in the room. When I first traveled to Israel some years ago, it was his stories that I thought of and that provided for me a sense of familiarity and comfort in a strange land. It is very clear that we are not encouraged as therapists to turn ourselves inside out publicly, or to pursue the answers to questions of communality and correction. As I write these words, I am torn between my affirmative answer to the Lovin' Spoonful's query and my great fear that these last words will invalidate what has come before in this book. It is not an accident that I have left these musings for the very end of the book. My hope is that these remarks will start a dialogue in which we can all pursue the best integrations, and stories, that we can tell.

References

Alexander, F. (1963). The dynamics of psychotherapy in the light of learning theory. *American Journal of Psychiatry, 120,* 440–448.

Alexander, F., & French, T. (1946). *Psychoanalytic therapy.* New York: Ronald Press.

Alford, B. A., & Norcross, J. C. (1991). Cognitive therapy as integrative therapy. *Journal of Psychotherapy Integration, 1,* 175–190.

Allen, D. M. (1993). Unified psychotherapy. In G. Stricker & J. R. Gold (Eds.), *Comprehensive handbook of psychotherapy integration* (pp. 125–138). New York: Plenum.

Andrews, J. D. (1989). Psychotherapy of depression: A self- confirmation model. *Psychological Review, 96,* 576–607.

Andrews, J. D. (1990). *The active self in psychotherapy: An integration of therapeutic styles.* Boston: Allyn & Bacon.

Andrews, J. D. (1993). The active self model: A paradigm for psychotherapy integration. In G. Stricker & J. R. Gold (Eds.), *Comprehensive handbook of psychotherapy integration* (pp. 165–186). New York: Plenum.

Applebaum, S. (1981). *Effecting change in psychotherapy.* New York: Jason Aronson.

Arkowitz, H. (1984). Historical perspective on the integration of psychoanalytic therapy and behavior therapy. In H. Arkowitz & S. Messer (Eds.), *Psychoanalytic therapy and behavioral therapy: Is integration possible?* (pp. 1–30). New York: Plenum.

Arkowitz, H. (1991). Introductory statement: Psychotherapy integration comes of age. *Journal of Psychotherapy Integration, 1,* 1–4.

Arkowitz, H., & Hannah, M. T. (1989). Cognitive, behavioral and psychodynamic therapies: Converging or diverging pathways to change? In A. Freeman, K. M. Simon, L. E. Beutler, & H. Arkowitz (Eds.), *Comprehensive handbook of cognitive therapy* (pp. 143–167). New York: Plenum.

Arkowitz, H., & Messer, S. (Eds.). (1984). *Psychoanalytic therapy and behavioral therapy: Is integration possible?* New York: Plenum.

Bandura, A. (1977). Self efficacy: Toward a unifying theory of behavior change. *Psychological Review, 84,* 191–215.

Bandura, A. (1982). Self efficacy mechanism in human agency. *American Psychologist, 37,* 122–147.

219

Bandura, A., & Walters, R. (1963). *Social learning and personality development.* New York: Holt, Rinehart and Winston.

Barkham, M., Shapiro, D. A., & Firth-Cozens, J. (1989). Personal questionnaire changes in prescriptive vs. exploratory psychotherapy. *British Journal of Clinical Psychology, 28,* 97–107.

Barnett, J. (1980). Cognitive repair in the treatment of the neuroses. *Journal of the American Academy of Psychoanalysis, 8,* 39–55.

Basch, M. F. (1985). Interpretation: Toward a developmental model. In A. Goldberg, (Ed.), *Progress in self psychology,* Vol. 1, (pp. 33-42). New York: Guilford Press.

Bateson, M. C. (1994). *Peripheral visions.* New York: HarperCollins.

Beck, A. T. (1976). *Cognitive therapy and the emotional disorders.* New York: New American Library.

Beck, A. T. (1991). Cognitive therapy as integrative therapy (commentary). *Journal of Psychotherapy Integration, 1,* 191–198.

Beck, A. T., & Emory, G. (1985). *Anxiety disorders and phobias.* New York: Guilford Press.

Beck, A. T., Freeman, A., & Associates (1989). *Cognitive therapy of personality disorders.* New York: Guilford Press.

Beck, A. T., Rush, A. J., Shaw, J., & Emory, G. (1979). *Cognitive therapy of depression.* New York: Guilford Press.

Becker, M. (1993). Organic disorders. In G. Stricker & J. R. Gold (Eds.), *Comprehensive handbook of psychotherapy integration* (pp. 353–364). New York: Plenum.

Beier, E. G. (1966). *The silent language of psychotherapy.* Chicago: Aldine.

Beitman, B. D. (1992). Integration through fundamental similarities and useful differences among the schools. In J. C. Norcross & M. R. Goldfried (Eds.), *Handbook of psychotherapy integration* (pp. 202–230). New York: Basic Books.

Bergin, A. E. (1968). Technique for improving desensitization via warmth, empathy, and emotional re-experiencing of hierarchy events. In R. Rubin & C. M. Franks (Eds.), *Advances in behavior therapy* (pp. 20-33). New York: Academic Press.

Berzonsky, M. D. (1992). A constructivist view of identity development: People as postpositivist self theorists. In J. Kroger (Ed.), *Discussions on ego identity* (pp. 169–203). Hillsdale, NJ: Erlbaum.

Beutler, L. E. (1983). *Eclectic psychotherapy: A systematic approach.* New York: Pergamon Press.

Beutler, L. E., & Consoli, A. J. (1992). Systematic eclectic psychotherapy. In J. C. Norcross & M. R. Goldfried (Eds.), *Handbook of psychotherapy integration* (pp. 264–299). New York: Basic Books.

Beutler, L. E., & Hodgson, A. B. (1993). Prescriptive psychotherapy. In G. Stricker & J. R. Gold (Eds.), *Comprehensive handbook of psychotherapy integration* (pp. 151–164). New York: Plenum.

Birk, L. (1970). Behavior therapy: Integration with dynamic therapy. *Behavior Therapy, 1,* 522–526.

Birk, L., & Brinkley-Birk, A. (1974). Psychoanalysis and behavior therapy. *American Journal of Psychiatry, 131,* 499-510.

Bohart, A. C. (1990). Psychotherapy integration from a client-centered perspective. In G. Lietaer, J. Rombauts, & R. Van Balen (Eds.), *Client-centered and experiential psychotherapy in the nineties* (pp. 481–506). Leuven, Belgium: Leuven University.

Bohart, A. C. (1991). Empathy in client-centered therapy. *Journal of Humanistic Psychology, 31,* 34–48.

Bohart, A. C. (1992). An integrative process model of psychopathology and psychotherapy. *Revista de Psicoterapia, 9,* 49–74.

Bohart, A. C. (1993). Experiencing: The basis of psychotherapy. *Journal of Psychotherapy Integration, 3,* 51–68.

Bohart, A. (1995). Mr. Lake. *Journal of Psychotherapy Integration, 5,* 119–130.

Bordin, E. S. (1994). Theory and research on the therapeutic working alliance: New directions. In A. O. Horvath & L. S. Greenberg (Eds.), *The working alliance: Theory, research and practice* (pp. 13–37). New York: Wiley.

Bowers, K. S. (1973). Situationism in psychology: An analysis and a critique. *Psychological Review, 80,* 307–336.

Bowlby, J. (1980). *Loss.* New York: Basic Books.

Brady, J. P. (1968). Psychotherapy by combined behavioral and dynamic approaches. *Comprehensive Psychiatry, 9,* 536–543.

Breuer, J., & Freud, S. (1895). *Studies on hysteria.* New York: Basic Books.

Bruner, J. (1990). Acts of meaning. Cambridge: Harvard University Press.

Bugenthal, J. F. T. (1965). *The search for authenticity.* New York: McGraw-Hill.

Bugenthal, J. F. T. (1981). *The search for authenticity* (2nd ed.). New York: Irvington.

Bugenthal, J. F. T., & Kleiner, R. (1993). Existential psychotherapies. In G. Stricker & J. R. Gold (Eds.), *Comprehensive handbook of psychotherapy integration* (pp. 101–112). New York: Plenum.

Butler, S. F., & Strupp, H. H. (1991). The role of affect in time limited dynamic psychotherapy. In J. D. Safran & L. S. Greenberg (Eds.), *Emotion, psychotherapy, and change* (pp. 83–112). New York: Guilford Press.

Carson, R. C. (1969). *Interaction concepts of personality.* Chicago: Aldine.

Cummings, N. (1993). Psychotherapy with substance abusers. In G. Stricker & J. R. Gold (Eds.), *Comprehensive handbook of psychotherapy integration* (pp. 337–352). New York: Plenum.

Curtis, R. C. (1993). Integrating social and clinical psychology. In G. Stricker & J. R. Gold (Eds.), *Comprehensive handbook of psychotherapy integration* (pp. 277–292). New York: Plenum.

Cushman, P. (1995). *Constructing the self, constructing America.* Boston: Addison-Wesley.

Daldrup, R. J., Beutler, L. E., Engle. D., & Greenberg, L. S. (1988). *Focused expressive psychotherapy.* New York: Guilford Press.

Daldrup, R. J., Engle, D., Holiman, M., & Beutler, L. E. (1991). The intensification and resolution of blocked affect in an experiential psychotherapy. *Journal of Integrative and Eclectic Psychotherapy, 10,* 329–339.

Davison, G. C. (1973). Counter control in behavior modification. In L. Hamerlynck, L. C. Handy, & E. J. Mash (Eds.), *Behavior change: Methodology, concepts, and practice* (pp. 323–356). Champaign, IL: Research Press.

Dollard, J., & Miller, N. E. (1950). *Personality and psychotherapy.* New York: McGraw-Hill.

Dowd, T. (1994). *Reactance in cognitive-behavior therapy.* Paper delivered at the fourth annual conference of the Society for the Exploration of Psychotherapy Integration, Buenos Aires, Argentina.

Dworkin, R. H., & Grzesiak, R. C. (1993). In G. Stricker & J. R. Gold (Eds.), *Comprehensive handbook of psychotherapy integration* (pp. 365–384). New York: Plenum.

Eissler, K. R. (1953). The effect of the structure of the ego on psychoanalytic technique. *Journal of the American Psychoanalytic Association, 1,* 104–143.

Ellis, A. (1984). Rational-emotive therapy. In R. J. Corsini, (Ed.), *Current psychotherapies* (3rd ed., pp. 331–378). Itaska, IL: Peacock.

Engle, D., Beutler, L. E., & Daldrup, R. J. (1991). Focused expressive psychotherapy: Treating blocked emotions. In J. D. Safran & L. S. Greenberg (Eds.), *Emotion, psychotherapy, and change* (pp. 161–196). New York: Guilford Press.

Eysenck, H. J. (1960). *Behavior therapy and the neuroses.* New York: Pergamon Press.

Feather, B. W., & Rhoades, J. W. (1972a) Psychodynamic behavior therapy: 1. Theory and rationale. *Archives of General Psychiatry, 26,* 496–502.

Feather, B. W., & Rhoades, J. W. (1972b). Psychodynamic behavior therapy: 2. Clinical aspects. *Archives of General Psychiatry, 26,* 503–511.

Fensterheim, H. (1993). Behavioral psychotherapy. In G. Stricker & J. Gold (Eds.), *The comprehensive handbook of psychotherapy integration* (pp. 73–86). New York: Plenum.

Ferenczi, S., & Rank, O. (1924). *Developments in psychoanalysis.* New York: Nervous and Mental Disease Publishing.

Fiedler, F. E. (1950). The concept of an ideal therapeutic relationship. *Journal of Consulting Psychology, 14,* 239–245.

Fisch, R. H., Weakland, J. H., & Segal, L. (1982). *The tactics of change.* San Francisco: Jossey-Bass.

Fischer, J. (1995). Uniformity myths in eclectic and integrative psychotherapy. *Journal of Psychotherapy Integration, 5,* 41–56.

Fishman, S. T., & Franks, C. M. (1992). The evolution of behavior therapy. In D. K. Freedheim (Ed.), *History of psychotherapy* (pp. 159–196). Washington, DC: American Psychological Association.

Fishman, S. T., & Lubetkin, B. S. (1983). Office practice of behavior therapy. In M. Hersen (Ed.), *Outpatient behavior therapy* (pp. 21–41). New York: Grune & Stratton.

Fitzpatrick, M. (1993). Adolescents. In G. Stricker & J. R. Gold (Eds.), *Comprehensive handbook of psychotherapy integration* (pp. 427–436). New York: Plenum.

Fodor, I. G. (1993). A feminist framework for integrative psychotherapy. In G. Stricker & J. R. Gold (Eds.), *Comprehensive handbook of psychotherapy integration* (pp. 217–236). New York: Plenum.

Frank, J. D. (1961). *Persuasion and healing.* Baltimore: Johns Hopkins University Press.

Frank, K. (1990). Action techniques in psychoanalysis. *Contemporary Psychoanalysis, 26,* 732–756.

Frank, K. (1993). Action, insight, and working through. *Psychoanalytic Dialogues, 3,* 40–55.

Frankl, V. E. (1960). Paradoxical intention: A logotherapeutic technique. *American Journal of Psychotherapy, 14,* 520–535.

Franklin, A. J., Carter, R. T., & Grace, C. (1993). An integrative approach to psychotherapy with Black/African Americans: The relevance of race and culture. In G. Stricker & J. R. Gold (Eds.), *Comprehensive handbook of psychotherapy integration* (pp. 465–482). New York: Plenum.

Franks, C. M. (1984). On conceptual and technical integration in psychoanalysis and behavior therapy: Two incompatible systems. In H. Arkowitz & S. Messer (Eds.), *Psychoanalytic therapy and behavioral therapy: Is integration possible?* (pp. 223–248). New York: Plenum.

French, T. M. (1933). Interrelations between psychoanalysis and the experimental work of Pavlov. *American Journal of Psychiatry, 89,* 1165–1203.

Freud, A. (1936). *The ego and the mechanisms of defense.* New York: International Universities Press.

Freud, S. (1894). Neuropsychoses of defense. In J. Strachey (Ed. and Trans.), *The standard edition of the complete psychological works of Sigmund Freud* (Vol. 3, pp. 43–68). London: Hogarth Press.

Freud, S. (1898). Further remarks on the neuropsychoses of defense. In J. Strachey (Ed. and Trans.), *The standard edition of the complete psychological works of Sigmund Freud* (Vol. 3, pp. 159–185). London: Hogarth Press.

Freud, S. (1900). The interpretation of dreams. In J. Strachey (Ed. and Trans.), *The standard edition of the complete psychological works of Sigmund Freud* (Vols. 4, 5.) London: Hogarth Press.

Freud, S. (1909). Notes upon a case of obsessional neurosis. In J. Strachey (Ed. and Trans.), *The standard edition of the complete psychological works of Sigmund Freud* (Vol. 10, pp. 153–318). London: Hogarth Press.

Freud, S. (1912). Dynamics of transference. In J. Strachey (Ed. and Trans.), *The standard edition of the complete psychological works of Sigmund Freud* (Vol. 12, pp. 97–108). London: Hogarth Press.

Freud, S. (1913). On beginning the treatment. In J. Strachey (Ed. and Trans.), *The standard edition of the complete psychological works of Sigmund Freud* (Vol. 12, pp. 121–149). London: Hogarth Press.

Freud; S. (1915). The unconscious. In J. Strachey (Ed. and Trans.), *The standard edition of the complete psychological works of Sigmund Freud* (Vol. 14, pp. 159–215). London: Hogarth Press.

Fried, E. (1983). *The courage to change.* New York: Norton.

Fromm, E. (1955). *The sane society.* New York: Henry Holt.

Fromm-Reichmann, R. (1950). *Principles of intensive psychotherapy.* Chicago: University of Chicago Press.

Garfield, S. L. (1980). *Psychotherapy: An eclectic approach.* New York: Wiley.

Garfield, S. L. (1992). Eclectic psychotherapy: A common factors approach. In J. C. Norcross & M. R. Goldfried (Eds.), *Handbook of psychotherapy integration* (pp. 169–201). New York: Basic Books.

Gaston, L., Goldfried, M. R., Greenberg, L. S., Horvath, A. O., Raue, P. J., & Watson, J. (1995). The therapeutic alliance in psychodynamic, cognitive-behavioral, and experiential therapies. *Journal of Psychotherapy Integration, 5,* 1–26.

Gendlin, E. (1979) *Focusing.* New York: Basic Books.

Gendlin, E. (1984). The client's client: The edge of awareness. In R. F. Levant & J. M. Shlein (Eds.), *Client-centered therapy and the person centered approach* (pp. 76–107). New York: Praeger.

Gill, M. M. (1982). *Analysis of transference* (Vol. 1). New York: International Universities Press.

Gill, M. (1994). *Psychoanalysis in transition.* New York: Basic Books.

Glass, C. G., & Arnkoff, D. B. (1992). Behavior therapy. In D. K. Freedheim (Ed.), *History of psychotherapy* (pp. 587–628). Washington, DC: American Psychological Association.

Gold, J. R. (1980). *A retrospective study of the behavior therapy experience.* Unpublished doctoral dissertation, Adelphi University.

Gold, J. R. (1990a). Culture, history, and psychotherapy integration. *Journal of Integrative and Eclectic Psychotherapy, 9,* 41–48.

Gold, J. R. (1990b). The integration of psychoanalytic, interpersonal, and cognitive approaches in the psychotherapy of borderline and narcissistic disorders. *Journal of Integrative and Eclectic Psychotherapy, 9,* 49–68.

Gold, J. R. (1992). An integrative-systemic approach to severe psychopathology in children and adolescents. *Journal of Integrative and Eclectic Psychotherapy, 11,* 67–78.

Gold, J. R. (1993a). An integrative approach to anxiety disorders. In G. Stricker and J. R. Gold (Eds.), *Comprehensive handbook of psychotherapy integration* (pp. 293–302). New York: Plenum.

Gold, J. R. (1993b). The socio-historical context of integrative therapy. In G. Stricker and J. R. Gold (Eds.), *Comprehensive handbook of psychotherapy integration* (pp. 3–8). New York: Plenum.

Gold, J. R. (1993c). The therapeutic interaction in psychotherapy integration. In G. Stricker and J. R. Gold (Eds.), *Comprehensive handbook of psychotherapy integration* (pp. 525–533). New York: Plenum.

Gold, J. R. (1994). When the patient does the integrating: Lessons for theory and practice. *Journal of Psychotherapy Integration, 4,* 133–154.

Gold, J. R. (1995). The role of process oriented therapy in an outcome oriented psychology and society. *Applied and Preventive Psychology, 4,* 61–74.

Gold, J. R., & Stricker, G. (1993). Psychotherapy integration with personality disorders. In G. Stricker & J. R. Gold (Eds.), *Comprehensive handbook of psychotherapy integration* (pp. 323–336). New York: Plenum.

Gold, J. R., & Wachtel, P. L. (1993). Cyclical psychodynamics. In G. Stricker & J. R. Gold (Eds.), *Comprehensive handbook of psychotherapy integration* (pp. 59–72). New York: Plenum.

Goldfried, M. R. (1980). Toward the delineation of therapeutic change principles. *American Psychologist, 35,* 991–999.

Goldfried, M. R. (1982). On the history of therapeutic integration. *Behavior Therapy, 13,* 572–593.

Goldfried, M. R. (1983). A behavior therapist looks at rapprochement. *Journal of Humanistic Psychology, 23,* 97–107.

Goldfried, M. R. (1991). Transtheoretical ingredients in therapeutic change. In R. C. Curtis & G. Stricker (Eds.), *How people change* (pp. 29–37). New York: Plenum.

Goldfried, M. R. (1994). *Cognitive-affective behavior therapy* (Video). Washington, DC: American Psychological Association.

Goldfried, M. R. (1995). *From cognitive behavior therapy to psychotherapy integration.* New York: Springer.

Goldfried, M. R., & Davison, G. (1976). *Clinical behavior therapy.* New York: Holt.

Goldfried, M. R., & Davison, G. (1994). *Clinical behavior therapy* (expanded ed.). New York: Holt.

Goldfried, M. R., & Newman, C. (1992). A history of psychotherapy integration. In J. C. Norcross & M. R. Goldfried (Eds.), *Handbook of psychotherapy integration* (pp. 46–93). New York: Basic Books.

Greenberg, J., & Mitchell, S. (1983). *Object relations in psychoanalytic theory.* Cambridge: Harvard University Press.

Greenberg, L. E. (1992). Process diagnosis of levels of emotional processing. *Journal of Psychotherapy Integration, 2,* 19–24.

Greenberg, L. E., & Rhodes, R. H. (1991). Emotion in the psychotherapy process. In R. C. Curtis & G. Stricker (Eds.), *How people change* (pp. 39–58). New York: Plenum.

Greenberg, L. E., Rice, L., & Elliot, R. (1993). *Process-experiential therapy: Facilitating emotional change.* New York: Guilford Press.

Greenberg, L. E., & Safran, J. D. (1984). Integrating affect and cognition: A perspective on the process of change. *Cognitive Therapy and Research, 8,* 559–578.

Grencavage, L. M., & Norcross, J. C. (1990). Where are the commonalties among the therapeutic common factors? *Professional Psychology: Research and Practice, 21,* 372–378.

Guidano, V. F. (1987). *Complexity of the self.* New York: Guilford Press.

Guidano, V. F. (1991). Affective change events in a cognitive therapy systems approach. In J. D. Safran & L. S. Greenberg (Eds.), *Emotion, psychotherapy, and change* (pp. 50–80). New York: Guilford Press.

Guidano, V. F., & Liotti, G. (1983). *Cognitive processes and the emotional disorders.* New York: Guilford Press.

Hayes, A. M., & Newman, C. F. (1993). Depression: An integrative perspective. In G. Stricker & J. R. Gold (Eds.), *Comprehensive handbook of psychotherapy integration* (pp. 303–322). New York: Plenum.

Healy, B. J. (1993). Psychotherapy and religious experience: Integrating psychoanalytic psychotherapy with Christian moral experience. In G. Stricker & J. R. Gold (Eds.), *Comprehensive handbook of psychotherapy integration* (pp. 267–276). New York: Plenum.

Heard, H. L., & Linehan, M. M. (1994). Dialectical behavior therapy: An integrative approach to the treatment of borderline personality disorder. *Journal of Psychotherapy Integration, 4,* 55–82.

Hellcamp, D. T. (1993). Serious mental disorders. In G. Stricker & J. R. Gold (Eds.), *Comprehensive handbook of psychotherapy integration* (pp. 385–400). New York: Plenum.

Herman, H. (1993). Imaginal dialogues in the self. *Journal of Personality, 61,* 207–236.

Holt, R. R. (1989). *Freud revisited.* New York: Guilford Press.

Horney, K. (1950). *Neurosis and human growth.* New York: Norton.

Horowitz, M. J. (1988). *Introduction to psychodynamics.* New York: Basic Books.

Horowitz, M. J. (1990). States, schemas, and control: General theories for psychotherapy integration. *Journal of Psychotherapy Integration, 2,* 85–102.

Hull, C. E. (1952). *A behavior system.* New Haven: Yale University Press.

Ischlondy, N. E. (1930). *Neuropsyche und hirnride: Physiologische grundlagen der tiefenpsychologie unter besonder berucksichting der psychoanalyse.* Berlin: Urban und Schwarzenberg. (Cited in Arkowitz, 1984.)

Izard, C. E. (1991). Perspectives on emotion in psychotherapy. In J. D. Safran & L. S. Greenberg (Eds.), *Emotion, psychotherapy, and change* (pp. 280–289). New York: Guilford Press.

Kanfer, F. H., & Schefft, B. K. (1988). *Guiding the process of therapeutic change.* Champaign, IL: Research Press.

Kelly, G. (1955). *The psychology of personal constructs* (Vol. 1). New York: Norton.

Kelly, G. (1963). *A theory of personality.* New York: Norton.

Kernberg, O. (1975). *Borderline conditions and pathological narcissism.* New York: Jason Aronson.

Kiesler, D. J. (1982). Interpersonal theory for personality and psychotherapy. In J. C. Anchin & D. J. Kiesler (Eds.), *Handbook of interpersonal psychotherapy* (pp. 3–24). New York: Pergamon Press.

Kirschner, S., & Kirschner, D. A. (1993). Couples and families. In G. Stricker & J. R. Gold (Eds.), *Comprehensive handbook of psychotherapy integration* (pp. 401–412). New York: Plenum.

Klein, G. S. (1971). *Psychoanalytic theory: an exploration of essentials.* New York: International Universities Press.

Kohlenberg, R. J., & Tsai, M. (1994). Functional analytic psychotherapy: A radical behavioral approach to treatment and integration. *Journal of Psychotherapy Integration, 4,* 175–202.

Kohut, H. (1977). *The restoration of the self.* New York: International Universities Press.

Kohut, H. (1980). *How does analysis cure?* New York: International Universities Press.

Kubie, L. (1934). Relation of the conditioned reflex to psychoanalytic technique. *Archives of Neurology and Psychiatry, 32,* 1137–1142.

Kuhn, T. S. (1962). *The structure of scientific revolution.* Chicago: University of Chicago Press.

Lambert, M. (1992). Psychotherapy outcome research: Implications for integrative and eclectic therapists. In J. C. Norcross & M. R. Goldfried, (Eds.), *Handbook of psychotherapy integration* (pp. 94–129). New York: Basic Books.

Lambert, M., & Bergin, A. E. (1994). The effectiveness of psychotherapy. In A. E. Bergin & S. L. Garfield (Eds.), *Handbook of psychotherapy and behavior change* (4th ed., pp. 143–189). New York: Wiley.

Lang, P. J. (1977). Imagery in therapy: An information processing analysis of fear. *Behavior Therapy, 8,* 862–886

Lang, P. J. (1979). A bio-informational theory of emotional imagery. *Psychophysiology, 16,* 495–512.

Lazarus, A. A. (1989). *The practice of multimodal therapy.* Baltimore: Johns Hopkins University Press.

Lazarus, A. A. (1992). Multimodal therapy: Technical eclecticism with minimal integration. In J. C. Norcross & M. R. Goldfried (Eds.), *Handbook of psychotherapy integration* (pp. 231–263). New York: Basic Books.

Lazarus, A. A. (1995). Different types of eclecticism and integration: Let's be aware of the dangers. *Journal of Psychotherapy Integration, 5,* 27–40.

Levant, R. F., & Shlein, J. W. (Eds.). (1984). *Client-centered therapy and the person-centered approach.* New York: Praeger.

Levenson, E. R. (1983). *The ambiguity of change.* New York: Basic Books.

Linehan, M. M. (1993). *Cognitive-behavioral treatment of borderline personality disorder.* New York: Guilford Press.

Llewelyn, S. P. (1988). Psychological therapy as viewed by clients and therapists. *British Journal of Clinical Psychology, 27,* 223–237.

Llewelyn, S. P., Elliot, R., Shapiro, D. A., & Hardy, G. (1988). Client perceptions of significant events in prescriptive and exploratory periods of individual therapy. *British Journal of Clinical Psychology, 27,* 105–114.

Loewald, H. (1960). On the therapeutic action of psychoanalysis. *International Journal of Psychoanalysis, 41,* 30–44.

London, P. (1964). *The modes and morals of psychotherapy.* New York: Holt, Rinehart and Winston.

Luborsky, L. (1984). *Principles of psychoanalytic psychotherapy: A manual for supportive-expressive treatment.* New York: Basic Books.

Luborsky, L. (1995). Are common factors across different psychotherapies the main explanation for the dodo bird verdict that "Everyone has won so all shall have prizes"? *Clinical Psychology: Science and Practice, 2,* 106–109.

Lyddon, W. J. (1992). Cognitive science and psychotherapy: An epistemic framework. In D. J. Stein & J. E. Young (Eds.), *Cognitive science and clinical disorders* (pp. 171–184). San Diego: Academic Press.

Mahler, M. S., Pine, F., & Bergman, A. (1975). *The psychological birth of the human infant.* New York: Basic Books.

Mahoney, M. J. (1991). *Human change processes.* New York: Basic Books.

Marks, I. M., & Gelder, M. G. (1966). Common ground between behavior therapy and psychodynamic methods. *British Journal of Medical Psychology, 39,* 11–23.

Marmor, J. (1971). Dynamic psychotherapy and behavior therapy: Are they reconcilable? *Archives of General Psychiatry, 24,* 22–28.

Maslow, A. H. (1954). *Motivation and personality.* New York: Harper & Row.

May, R. (1977). *The meaning of anxiety.* New York: Norton.

May, R., & Yalom, I. (1989). Existential therapy. In R. J. Corsini & D. Weddings (Eds.), *Current psychotherapies* (pp. 363–402). Itaska, IL: Peacock.

McCullough, L. (1993). An anxiety reduction modification of short term dynamic psychotherapy (STDP): A theoretical melting pot of treatment techniques. In G. Stricker & J. R. Gold (Eds.), *Comprehensive handbook of psychotherapy integration* (pp. 139–150). New York: Plenum.

McGuire, K. (1991). Affect in experiential and focusing psychotherapy. In J. D. Safran & L. S. Greenberg (Eds.), *Emotion, psychotherapy, and change* (pp. 227–254). New York: Guilford Press.

Menninger, K. (1958). *The theory of psychoanalytic technique.* New York: Basic Books.

Messer, S. (1992). A critical examination of belief structures in integrative and eclectic psychotherapy. In J. C. Norcross & M. R. Goldfried (Eds.), *Handbook of psychotherapy integration* (pp. 130–168). New York: Basic Books.

Messer, S., & Winokur, M. (1984). Ways of knowing and visions of reality in psychoanalytic therapy and behavior therapy. In H. Arkowitz & S. Messer (Eds.), *Psychoanalytic therapy and behavioral therapy: Is integration possible?* (pp. 63–100). New York: Plenum.

Mischel, W. (1973). Toward a cognitive social learning reconceptualization of personality. *Psychological Review, 80,* 252–283.

Mitchell, S. (1988). *Relational concepts in psychoanalysis.* Cambridge: Harvard University Press.

Mitchell, S. (1993). *Hope and dread in psychoanalysis.* New York: Basic Books.

Mowrer, O. H. (1953). *Psychotherapy: Theory and research.* New York: Ronald Press.

Newirth, J. W. (1995). *The Wizard of Oz or Sir Lancelot.* Paper presented at the annual meeting of the Division of Psychoanalysis, American Psychological Association, Los Angeles.

Niemeyer, R. (1993). Constructivism and the problem of psychotherapy integration. *Journal of Psychotherapy Integration, 3,* 133–158.

Niemeyer, R., & Feixas, G. (1990). Constructivist contributions to psychotherapy integration. *Journal of Integrative and Eclectic Psychotherapy, 9,* 4–20.

Norcross, J. C., & Goldfried, M. R. (Eds.). (1992). *Handbook of psychotherapy integration.* New York: Basic Books.

Norcross, J. C., & Newman, C. (1992). Psychotherapy integration: Setting the context. In J. C. Norcross & M. R. Goldfried (Eds.), *Handbook of psychotherapy integration* (pp. 47–83). New York: Basic Books.

Oatley, K. (1992). Integrative action of narrative. In D. J. Stein & J. E. Young (Eds.), *Cognitive science and clinical disorders* (pp. 151–172). San Diego: Academic Press.

O'Hara, M. M. (1984). Person centered gestalt: Toward a holistic synthesis. In R. F. Levant & J. W. Shlein (Eds.), *Client-centered therapy and the person centered approach* (pp. 256–270). New York: Praeger.

O'Leary, K. D., & Wilson, G. T. (1987). *Behavior therapy: Application and outcome.* Englewood Cliffs, NJ: Prentice-Hall.

Orlinsky, D. E., Grawe, K., & Parks, B. K. (1994). Process and outcome in psychotherapy—Noch einmal. In A. E. Bergin & S. L. Garfield (Eds.), *Handbook of psychotherapy and behavior change* (4th ed., pp. 270–378). New York: Wiley.

Orlinsky, D. E., & Howard, K. I. (1986). The psychological interior of psychotherapy: Explorations with the Therapy Session Report Questionnaire. In L. S. Greenberg & W. M. Pinsoff (Eds.), *The psychotherapeutic process: A research handbook* (pp. 477–501). New York: Guilford Press.

Oz, A. (1995). *Under this blazing light.* Cambridge, UK: Cambridge University Press.

Papouchis, N., & Passman, V. (1993). An integrative approach to the psychotherapy of the elderly. In G. Stricker & J. R. Gold (Eds.), *Comprehensive handbook of psychotherapy integration* (pp. 437–452). New York: Plenum.

Pascual-Leone, J. (1991). Emotions, development and psychotherapy: A dialectical-constructivistic perspective. In J. D. Safran & L. S. Greenberg (Eds.), *Emotion, psychotherapy, and change* (pp. 302–338). New York: Guilford Press.

Perls, F. (1973). *The gestalt approach: A eyewitness to therapy.* New York: Science and Behavior Books.

Perls, F., & Goodman, P., Hefferline, R. F., (1951). *Gestalt therapy.* New York: Julian Press.

Piaget, J. (1926). *The language and thought of the child* (Trans. M. Worden). New York: Harcourt, Brace.

Powell, D. H. (1988). Spontaneous insight associated with behavior therapy: The case of Rex. *Journal of Integrative and Eclectic Psychotherapy, 1,* 140–166.

Prochaska, J. O. (1984). *Systems of psychotherapy: A transtheoretical analysis* (2nd ed.). Homewood, IL: Dorsey.

Prochaska, J. O. (1995). Common problems: Common solutions. *Clinical Psychology: Science and Practice, 2,* 101–105.

Prochaska, J. O., & DiClemente, C. C. (1992a). Stages of change in the modification of problem behaviors. In M. Hersen, R. M. Eisler, & P. M. Miller (Eds.), *Progress in behavior modification* (Vol. 28, (pp. 262–289). Newberry, CA: Sage.

Prochaska, J. O., & DiClemente, C. C. (1992b). The transtheoretical approach. In J. C. Norcross & M. R. Goldfried (Eds.), *Handbook of psychotherapy integration* (pp 300–334). New York: Basic Books.

Rachman, S. (1981). The primacy of affect: Some theoretical implications. *Behaviour Research and Theory, 19,* 270–290.

Rachman, S. (1984). A reassessment of the "Primacy of Affect." *Cognitive Therapy and Research, 6,* 579–584.

Racker, H. (1968). *Transference and countertransference.* New York: International Universities Press.

Raskin, R. (1994). *Client centered therapy* (Video). Washington, DC: American Psychological Association.

Raskin, R., & Rogers, C. R. (1989). Person centered therapy. In R. J. Corsini & D. Weddings (Eds.), *Current psychotherapies* (pp. 155–196). Itaska, IL: Peacock.

Raue, P. J., & Goldfried, M. R. (1994). The therapeutic alliance in cognitive-behavior therapy. In A. O. Horvath & L. S. Greenberg (Eds.), *The working alliance: Theory, research and practice* (pp. 131–152). New York: Wiley.

Reeve, J., Inck, T., & Safran, J. (1993). Toward an integration of cognitive, interpersonal, and experiential approaches to psychotherapy. In G. Stricker & J. R. Gold (Eds.),

Comprehensive handbook of psychotherapy integration (pp. 113–124). New York: Plenum.

Reich, W. (1949). *Character analysis*. New York: Noonday Press.

Rhodes, J. M. (1984). Relationships between psychodynamic and behavior therapies. In H. Arkowitz & S. Messer, (Eds.), *Psychoanalytic therapy and behavioral therapy: Is integration possible?* (pp. 195–212). New York: Plenum.

Rice, L. N. (1984). Client tasks in client-centered therapy. In R. F. Levant & J. W. Shlein (Eds.), *Client-centered therapy and the person-centered approach* (pp. 182–202). New York: Praeger.

Rice, L. N., & Greenberg, L. S. (1991). Two affective change events in client centered therapy. In J. D. Safran & L. S. Greenberg, (Eds.)., *Emotion, psychotherapy, and change* (pp. 197–226). New York: Guilford Press.

Rice, L. N. & Greenberg, L. S. (1992). Humanistic approaches to psychotherapy. In D. K. Freedheim (Ed.), *History of psychotherapy* (pp. 337–363). Washington, DC: American Psychological Association.

Rogers, C. R. (1957). The necessary and sufficient conditions of therapeutic personality change. *Journal of Consulting Psychology, 21*, 95–103.

Rogers, C. R. (1959). The essence of psychotherapy. *Annals of Psychotherapy, 1*, 51–57.

Rogers, C. R. (1961). *On becoming a person*. Boston: Houghton Mifflin.

Rosenzweig, S. (1936). Some implicit common factors in diverse methods in psychotherapy. *American Journal of Orthopsychiatry, 6*, 412–415.

Rubin, J. B. (1993). Psychoanalysis and Buddhism: Towards an integration. In G. Stricker & J. R. Gold (Eds.), *Comprehensive handbook of psychotherapy integration* (pp. 249–266). New York: Plenum.

Ryle, A. (1990). *Cognitive-analytic therapy: Active participation in change*. Chichester, England: Wiley.

Ryle, A., & Low, J. (1993). Cognitive analytic therapy. In G. Stricker & J. R. Gold (Eds.), *Comprehensive handbook of psychotherapy integration* (pp. 87–100). New York: Plenum.

Safran, J. D., & Greenberg, L. S. (Eds.). (1991). *Emotion, psychotherapy, and change*. New York: Guilford Press.

Safran, J. D., & Segal, Z. D. (1990). *Interpersonal processes in cognitive therapy*. New York: Basic Books.

Salter, A. (1949). *Conditioned reflex therapy*. New York: Creative Age.

Sandler, J. (1960). The background of safety. *International Journal of Psychoanalysis, 41*, 352–356.

Sass, L. (1988). Humanism, hermeneutics, and the concept of the human subject. In S. Messer, L. Sass, & R. Woolfolk (Eds.), *Hermeneutics and psychological theory* (pp. 250–279). New Brunswick, NJ: Rutgers University Press.

Schacht, T. (1984). The varieties of integrative experience. In H. Arkowitz, & S. Messer, (Eds.), *Psychoanalytic therapy and behavioral therapy: Is integration possible?* (pp. 107–132). New York: Plenum.

Sears, R. R. (1944). Experimental analysis of psychoanalytic phenomena. In J. McV. Hunt (Ed.), *Personality and the behavior disorders* (pp. 191–206). New York: Ronald Press.

Shlein, J. M. (1984). A countertheory of transference. In R. F. Levant & J. M. Shlein (Eds.), *Client-centered therapy and the person centered approach* (pp. 176–207). New York: Praeger.

Shapiro, A. K., & Morris, L. A. (1978). The placebo effect in medical and psychological therapies. In S. L. Garfield & A. E. Bergin (Eds.), *Handbook of psychotherapy and behavior change* (2nd ed., pp. 369–410). New York: Wiley.

Shapiro, D. (1965). *Neurotic styles.* New York: Basic Books.

Shapiro, D. (1989). *Psychotherapy of neurotic character.* New York: Basic Books.

Shapiro, D. A. (1981). Comparative credibility of treatment rationales: Three tests of expectancy theory. *British Journal of Clinical Psychology, 21,* 111–122.

Shapiro, D. A. , Barkham, M., Reynolds, S., Hardy, G., & Stiles, W. B. (1992). Prescriptive and exploratory psychotherapies: Toward and integration based on the assimilation model. *Journal of Psychotherapy Integration, 2,* 253–272.

Schafer, R. (1976). *A new language for psychoanalysis.* New Haven: Yale University Press.

Shoben, E. J. (1949). Psychotherapy as a problem in learning theory. *Psychological Bulletin, 46,* 366–392.

Simkin, J. S., & Yontef, G. M. (1984). Gestalt therapy. In J. C. Raymond (Ed.), *Current psychotherapies* (pp. 323–246). Itaska IL: Peacock.

Singer, E. (1965). *Key concepts in psychotherapy.* New York: Basic Books.

Sloane, R. B. (1969). The converging paths of psychotherapy and behavior therapy. *American Journal of Psychiatry, 125,* 877–885.

Sollod, R. N. (1993). Integrating spiritual healing approaches and techniques into psychotherapy. In G. Stricker & J. R. Gold (Eds.), *Comprehensive handbook of psychotherapy integration* (pp. 237–248). New York: Plenum.

Spence, D. (1982). *Narrative truth and historical truth.* New York: Norton.

Stampfl, T. G., & Levis, D. J. (1967). Essentials of implosive therapy: A learning theory based psychodynamic behavioral therapy. *Journal of Abnormal Psychology, 72,* 496–503.

Stampfl, T. G., & Levis, D. J. (1976). Implosive therapy: A behavioral therapy? In J. Spence, R. Carson, & J. Thibaut (Eds.), *Behavioral approaches to therapy* (pp. 189–210). Morristown, NJ: General Learning Press.

Stein, D. J., & Young, J. E. (Eds.). (1992). *Cognitive science and clinical disorders* (pp. 171–184). San Diego: Academic Press.

Stern, D. (1985). *The interpersonal world of the infant.* New York: Basic Books.

Stiles, W. B., Barkham, M., Shapiro, D. A., & Firth-Cozens, J. (1992). Treatment order and thematic continuity between contrasting psychotherapies: Exploring an implication of the assimilation model. *Psychotherapy Research, 2,* 112–124.

Strachey, J. (1934). The nature of the therapeutic action of psychoanalysis. *International Journal of Psychoanalysis, 15,* 127–159.

Stricker, G., & Gold, J. R. (Eds.). (1993). *Comprehensive handbook of psychotherapy integration.* New York: Plenum.

Strupp, H. H. (1971). On the basic ingredients of psychotherapy. *Journal of Consulting and Clinical Psychology, 41,* 1–8.

Strupp, H. H., & Binder, J. (1984). *Psychotherapy in a new key.* New York: Basic Books.

Strupp, H. H., Hadley, S., & Gomes-Schwartz, B. (1977). *Psychotherapy for better or worse.* New York: Aronson.

Strupp, H. H., Wallach, M. S., & Wogan, M. (1964). Psychotherapy experience in retrospect: A questionnaire study of former patients and therapists. *Psychological Monographs, 78.*

Sullivan, H. S. (1953). *The interpersonal theory of psychiatry.* New York: Norton.

Sweet, A. A. (1985). The therapeutic relationship in behavior therapy. *Clinical Psychology Review, 8,* 253–272.

Vaillant, G. (1993). *The wisdom of the ego.* Cambridge: Harvard University Press.

Wachtel, E. F., & Wachtel, P. L. (1986). *Family dynamics in individual therapy.* New York: Guilford Press.

Wachtel, P. L. (1977). *Psychoanalysis and behavior therapy: Toward an integration.* New York: Basic Books.

Wachtel, P. L. (1985). Integrative psychodynamic therapy. In S. Lynn & J. Garske (Eds.), *Contemporary psychotherapies* (pp. 148–179). Columbus, OH: Merrill.

Wachtel, P. L. (1989). *The poverty of affluence.* Philadelphia: New Society.

Wachtel, P. L. (1991). From eclecticism to synthesis: Toward a more seamless psychotherapeutic integration. *Journal of Psychotherapy Integration, 1,* 43–54.

Wachtel, P. L. (1993). *Therapeutic communication.* New York: Guilford Press.

Wachtel, P. L., & McKinney, M. K. (1992). Cyclical psychodynamics and integrative psychodynamic therapy. In J. C. Norcross & M. R. Goldfried (Eds.), *Handbook of psychotherapy integration* (pp. 335–372). New York: Basic Books.

Watson, J. C., & Greenberg, L. S. (1994). The alliance in experiential therapy: Enacting the relationship conditions. In A. O. Horvath & L. S. Greenberg (Eds.), *The working alliance: Theory, research, and practice* (pp. 153–172). New York: Wiley.

Weinberger, J. (1993). Common factors in psychotherapy. In G. Stricker & J. R. Gold (Eds.), *Comprehensive handbook of psychotherapy integration* (pp. 43–58). New York: Plenum.

Weinberger, J. (1995). Common factors aren't so common. *Clinical Psychology: Science and Practice, 2,* 45–69.

Weiss, J. (1994). *How psychotherapy works.* New York: Guilford Press.

Weiss, J., & Sampson, H. (1986). *The psychoanalytic process.* New York: Guilford Press.

Weitzman, B. (1967). Behavior therapy and psychotherapy. *Psychological Review, 74,* 300–317.

Westerman, M. A. (1993), A hermeneutic approach to integration: Psychotherapy within the circle of practical activity. In G. Stricker & J. R. Gold (Eds.), *Comprehensive handbook of psychotherapy integration* (pp. 187–217). New York: Plenum.

Weston, D. (1988). Transference and information processing. *Clinical Psychology Review, 8,* 161–179.

White, M., & Epson, D. (1990). *Narrative means to therapeutic ends.* New York: Norton.

Winnicott, D. W. (1971). *The maturational processes and the facilitating environment.* New York: International Universities Press.

Wolf, E. (1988). *Treating the self.* New York: Guilford Press.

Wolfe, B. E. (1992a). Integrative psychotherapy of the anxiety disorders. In J. C. Norcross & M. R. Goldfried (Eds.), *Handbook of psychotherapy integration* (pp. 373–401). New York: Basic Books.

Wolfe, B. E. (1992b). Self experiencing and the integrative treatment of the anxiety disorders. *Journal of Psychotherapy Integration, 2,* 29–44.

Wolpe, J. (1958). *Psychotherapy through reciprocal inhibition.* Stanford, CA: Stanford University Press.

Wolpe, J. (1984). Behavior therapy according to Lazarus. *American Psychologist, 39,* 1326–1327.

Wolstein, B. (1990). Five empirical psychoanalytic methods. *Contemporary Psychoanalysis, 26,* 237–256.

Yalom, I. (1981). *Existential psychotherapy.* New York: Basic Books.

Yontef, G. (1969). *A review of the practice of gestalt therapy.* Los Angeles: Trident.

Yontef, G. (1989). The future of gestalt therapy. *The Gestalt Journal, 4,* 67–79.

Young, J. E. (1992). *Cognitive therapy for personality disorders: A schema based approach.* New York: Guilford Press.

Zajonc, R. (1980). Feeling and thinking: Preferences need no inferences. *American Psychologist, 35,* 151–175.

Index